5/18

Hac
Get stronger,
live longer!
Lisa

MW01504369

What People Are Saying About
Lisa Teresi Harris and *Building Your Enduring Fitness*

"Better health begins with awareness, knowledge, and a formula to get you to where you want to be. This book has it all! I appreciate the author's common sense approach to a healthier lifestyle because her prescription is not extreme in any manner. It is comprised of simple modifications and guidelines that fit nicely with modern day living."

— Dr. Richard B. Greene, The IronMan Business Coach and Author of *The 10 Commandments of Peak Performance*

"In *Building Your Enduring Fitness*, Lisa Harris reveals the truths about aging and what we can do to stay healthy and active. Most diseases can be prevented if we make the right food and exercise choices. Whether you're young and healthy, middle-aged, or over eighty, you'll find nuggets of hope and health in these pages."

— Nicole Gabriel, Author of *Finding Your Inner Truth* and *Healing Your Dog Naturally*

"Lisa helps you step into a self-leadership role in your own wellness. I love that her book helps you become empowered in your health so you can *shine*!"

— Rebecca Hall Gruyter, Women's Empowerment Leader, CEO/Owner of RHG Media Productions and Your Purpose Driven Practice

"Lisa Harris proves that the age-old adage is true: 'You're only as old as you think you are.' Even centenarians can live youthful lives, and Lisa shows how someday you can join their club. From fitness tips to the lowdown on how to prevent diseases, *Building Your Enduring Fitness* is packed with the stuff that will make you feel young and strong again."

— Patrick Snow, Publishing Coach and Best-Selling Author of *Creating Your Own Destiny* and *Boy Entrepreneur*

"Lisa Harris gets it! There's just too much conflicting information out there about fitness and nutrition for Baby Boomers and older adults. She takes all the scientific jargon and distills it down to useful tips for you to follow."

— Tara Borghese, Author/Speaker and creator of "Moments with Miley"

"This book made me want to get up and move so much that it was hard for me to sit and finish reading it. The fact, as Lisa Harris explains, is that if we just keep moving we can do a lot to forestall the aging process. If you need motivation, then *Building Your Enduring Fitness* definitely fits the bill!"

— Tyler R. Tichelaar, PhD and Award-Winning Author of *Narrow Lives* and *Haunted Marquette*

"I am so glad I found this book! In *Building Your Enduring Fitness*, Lisa Harris presents facts and processes to help me rebuild my body. Suffering from an arthritic knee, I am unable to do what I use to do and the weight is piling on. Lisa touched on everything I need in order to move forward to a healthier lifestyle. This book couldn't have come at a better time. What are you waiting for? Get this book now so you can live your best!"

— Alicia White, Founder, Back of the Room Productions

"At last, a guide that is practical, easy to read, and based on the latest in scientific information to help you truly take charge of your health and reshape your future well-being!"

— Patti Cotton, CEO, Cotton Group

BUILDING YOUR
ENDURING
FITNESS

*Age-Defying
Strategies That
Boost Your
Vitality*

LISA TERESI HARRIS, MS, RD, ACE-CPT

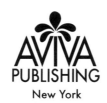

AVIVA
PUBLISHING
New York

Building Your Enduring Fitness: Age-Defying Strategies That Boost Your Vitality

Published by:
Aviva Publishing
Lake Placid, NY
(518) 523-1320
www.AvivaPubs.com

Address all inquiries to:
Lisa Teresi Harris
(951) 533-2612
lisa@enduringfitness4u.com
BuildingYourEnduringFitness.com

Disclaimer: Stories in this book are based upon real-life situations, but names have been changed to protect individuals' privacy.

ISBN: 978-1-947937-23-9
Library of Congress Control Number: 2018900217

Editor: Tyler Tichelaar/Superior Book Productions
Cover Designer: Nicole Gabriel/Angel Dog Productions
Interior Book Layout: Nicole Gabriel/Angel Dog Productions
Author Photo: Su Loew

Every attempt has been made to source all quotes properly.
Printed in the United States of America
First Edition
2 4 6 8 10 12

DEDICATION

To my mother, Jean M. Teresi. As long as I can remember, your advice was: "If you work hard enough, you can accomplish anything." And here I am. Your love and encouragement were my inspiration, the reason I went back to school at fifty-nine and started my second career.

To my father, Joseph A. Teresi. You left us way too early. I wish you could have lived longer to enjoy your grandchildren and great-grandchildren. I admired your love of family and your untiring work ethic, and I owe my perseverance, level-headedness, and thriftiness to you.

To my husband, Terry, thank you for sticking with me through all my crazy ideas. You've been my partner and best friend for more than thirty years. Your love and support have been my anchor, and believe me, I've needed that stability often.

To my daughters, Jackie Bailey and Lindsay Harris. You've become pretty cool young ladies. Thanks for encouraging me and teaching this old gal about new technology and social media.

And to my grandchildren, Elly, Keegan, and Loghan, you're a huge part of my big "why"!

With love, I dedicate this book to you all!

ACKNOWLEDGMENTS

Thanks to all the following, without whom my second career and this book would not have been possible:

Dorothy Chen Maynard, whose connections in 2013 led me everywhere I've been since then; Fabio Comana, who convinced me I might earn a living as a fitness professional; business coaches Patti Cotton, Jacqui Dobens, Margie Geyser, Jill Lublin, and Katrina Sawa; Michelle Skiljan and the brilliant mentors at the Inland Empire Women's Business Center; and Brent Williams for my first job as a personal trainer.

Fellow members of the Live Big MasterMind group, Business Women's Network of Temecula Valley, Professional Women's Roundtable, and Professional Women's Toastmasters for their support and guidance.

My book coach Patrick Snow; designer Nicole Gabriel; and editor Tyler Tichelaar.

My fabulous clients and exercise class participants.

All of my friends and family, for the love and support over the years.

DISCLAIMER

This book is written as a source of information only. The information contained in this book should by no means be considered a substitute for the advice of a qualified medical professional, who should always be consulted before beginning any new diet, exercise, or other health program. All efforts have been made to ensure the accuracy of the information contained in this book as of the date published. While the author has no control over websites she does not operate, all links were active at the time of research. The publisher and the author disclaim liability for any adverse effects that may occur as a result of applying the methods suggested in this book.

CONTENT

Special Reports

TURNING BACK THE HANDS OF TIME

How does your future wellness look? In answering this question, I hope you're not a "typical" Baby Boomer or older adult, accepting that your best days have passed you by.

Let's take a quick look at your current health conditions. Do any of the following statements describe you? Your doctor recently threw the diagnosis "prediabetes" at you, and you have no idea what to do! Your best friend just died at age forty-eight from a heart attack, and you're wondering whether you're next! You've heard the latest statistics about Alzheimer's disease, and they scare you to death! You know you need to lose weight, but you're stuck with extra pounds! You're overwhelmed with all the health information online and don't know where to turn for advice!

Are you concerned you won't be able to live out your life with quality, strength, and independence? Are your muscles getting flabbier and weaker? Do you see chronic diseases—diabetes, cancer, heart disease, dementia—as an inevitable part of your future? Are you afraid of falling and not being able to get up? Do you worry you won't live long enough to see your grandchildren get married?

I know how you feel! At age forty-two, I received a diagnosis that threw my life into a tailspin. I'd been experiencing strange symptoms—double vision, droopy eyelids. Luckily, my doctor acted quickly and ordered a simple blood test. The result—*myasthenia gravis*, Latin for "grave muscle weakness."

There I was with a fabulous marriage, two beautiful young daughters, a promising career—and an incurable autoimmune neuromuscular disorder! After the appropriate feeling-sorry-for-myself period and attendance at a few support meetings, I decided I wasn't going to let this new label define my life. My husband and I chose the best course of action; I started on immunosuppressants and had surgery to remove my thymus gland.

I knew how to eat for my recovery (and beyond) and gradually regained my strength. A few years later, I stepped into a gym and did what was previously unthinkable—I started lifting weights. Today, nobody would guess I have a "muscle weakness" disease.

But life wasn't done with me in terms of chronic disease. Genetics and "wear and tear" caught up with me this year in the form of bone-on-bone arthritis in my left hip. No longer able to count on walking as my primary mode of cardiovascular exercise, I knew I had to think outside the box. I asked myself what I would tell my clients when pain causes them to give up on movement. The answer: Find another activity that doesn't hurt! I've now turned my light-weight road bike into a convenient stationary bicycle that sits outside my kitchen, ready for me to use at any time of day, in any weather!

In this book, I'll take *you* on a self-leadership journey to build *your* optimum health. You'll learn to find your purpose or "big why" to keep you motivated while making lifestyle changes. You'll identify support systems—family, friends, and professionals—to whom you can turn in good times and bad. You'll learn the importance of movement and how to incorporate it effortlessly into your life. I'll demonstrate the age-defying benefits of a plant-based diet and show you how to begin nudging yourself in that direction.

Then you'll face down chronic diseases. Whether it's arthritis, cancer, diabetes, heart disease, or dementia and Alzheimer's, you'll learn strategies to live the healthy, quality life you seek. You'll grasp the health-sustaining need for optimal water and protein intake. I'll show you how to take on your fear of falling and how to get up if you do go down. And because you don't always live in a perfect world where you prepare your own healthful food, you'll learn tips for successful dining away from home.

If you apply the strategies, knowledge, and techniques in this book to your own wellness, then you will achieve what my title and subtitle promise, *Building Your Enduring Fitness: Age-Defying Strategies That Boost Your Vitality.* You'll have tips to outsmart Mother Nature and turn back the hands of time. You'll know where to look for information you can rely on to live your life with the quality and self-sufficiency you desire.

But why trust me with your wellness journey? First of all, you've seen that I've been there—I am one of you, a Baby Boomer striving to live my best life with chronic disease. I've been a registered dietitian since the 1970s and a certified personal trainer with a specialty in senior fitness since 2013. The blending of these two fields of expertise is important for you because it's outside the scope of practice for dietitians to give specific fitness advice, and, likewise, personal trainers are not equipped to treat medical conditions through nutrition. But with both backgrounds, I am uniquely qualified to offer wellness advice in the areas of fitness/ exercise *and* nutrition/food.

In 2014, I started my business, Enduring Fitness 4U, providing fitness training and nutrition coaching for Baby Boomers and older adults. I've helped hundreds of people over age fifty to increase their fitness levels. I've won entrepreneurial awards and written health-related articles for magazines, including *Shape* and *Men's Fitness*, newspapers, and more than 150 blogs. I've spoken at numerous universities and organizations, and been interviewed on podcasts and radio shows.

But still, I don't know everything. In the exercise and nutrition fields, information is constantly changing, and that means I'm always learning. You know what I mean. Eggs are bad for you; eggs are good for you. Carbs will send your health down the drain; carbs are important for weight loss and gut health. Lifting weight is good, but high-intensity intervals are better. And what works for me won't necessarily work for you. My clients are constantly teaching me new ways to approach their problems. Readers of my blogs ask the questions that keep me researching for the best answers. And you can help me learn more with your responses to this book.

I understand why you're standing there reading this introduction. I get that your waistband is a little tighter than it was last year, that your A1C level just bounced into the prediabetes stage, that you're worried about falling or losing your mental capacity.

Lifestyle changes are extremely difficult to make and to maintain. You see conflicting information all the time—online, on billboards, through radio and television ads, and in interviews. But I know you want to start changing your life; that's why this book caught your attention. It's okay. I believe in you and your ability to begin turning your health around.

I want to be with you during this journey. I want to be your coach and a shoulder you can lean on while taking on these life-changing strategies. I'll provide you with resources and answer your questions to help you overcome the challenges that have stopped you in the past. And I challenge you to begin your life makeover today!

Are you ready to begin? Are you ready to take a good look at your current health and lifestyle choices? Can you see the energetic, strong person you yearn to become? Are you ready to step out of your comfort zone so you can finally realize wellness success? Will you set attainable goals and achieve them? If so, that's fabulous! Let's get started and make this journey together! Now is your time. (You're not getting any younger.) So lace up your walking shoes, clean out your refrigerator, and let's go!

Lisa Harris

CHAPTER 1

TAKING ON THE SELF-LEADERSHIP ROLE IN YOUR WELLNESS

"The first wealth is health."

— Ralph Waldo Emerson

SUDDENLY, YOU'RE FEELING OLD

Just who is that person staring back at you in the mirror? What's going on with your face, your muscles, your posture? One day, you look and feel great; the next day, you're noticing less strength and energy, and you wonder when your pants started shrinking.

Eventually, it happens to all of us—the mental picture you carry around of yourself and the image in the mirror don't jive any more.

You can blame it on Mother Nature—she's just not kind to us as we age. Consider the following problems that will occur if you don't intervene:

- By the time you reach seventy or eighty, you'll lose a significant amount of muscle mass and strength.

- Loss of muscle leads to a decreased ability to live independently. And the relative percentage of body fat increases, bringing with it increased risk of chronic diseases.

- Weak muscles and bones lead to falls. Every twenty-nine minutes, an older adult dies from a fall.[1]

- The brain loses volume, cells, and connections with age. These problems are related to dementias, including Alzheimer's.

So if you do nothing, you'll end up in trouble. Like some of my clients, you might have medical issues that weaken your legs. You drop into a comfy chair for a year or two, and when you've had enough sitting, you simply can't get up. Or, like my mother-in-law, you'll lie in your hospital bed, awaiting open-heart surgery and wondering how you got there. It's a gradual process, but it happens.

Despite the challenges that accompany aging, most of us would like to live to 100, according to a recent survey of more than 4,000 Americans.[2] But that longevity balances on a double-edged sword: We want to live longer, but we are concerned about losing mental or physical capabilities, becoming a burden, being alone, or experiencing financial problems. In fact, 41 percent of financial planners say their clients' top concern about retirement is running out of money because of decreasing income and fear of escalating healthcare costs.[3]

LIVE OUT YOUR LIFE WITH DIGNITY

I saw these concerns very clearly about ten years ago when I was visiting my mother. Mom was living in an independent care facility in Colorado, and I stayed with her for about a week. As I joined Mom during meals and got to know the lovely ladies she lived and dined with, I started to notice a pattern. Their conversations always revolved around two topics: what was on the menu for this meal and the next, and what the residents were afraid of. And their fears were these: falling and getting pneumonia. Each one knew that if either of those incidents occurred, she would have to leave her home. She feared she might become a burden to her family or never return to her friends.

I came back to California with an epiphany—many of Mom's friends were simply waiting to move on to the next level of care. They felt their declining health was inevitable.

At that moment, I realized everybody, no matter what his or her age, wants to live out life with as much independence and dignity as possible.

So at fifty-seven, having been a registered dietitian and involved in healthcare for more than thirty years, I went back to school to become a certified personal trainer. Then I started my business, Enduring Fitness 4U, providing nutrition counseling and strength training for people over fifty.

I now know, without a doubt, that while we all grow old, it is possible to control how and when we age. In fact, many of the conditions we associate with old age (including Alzheimer's) are *not* a normal part of aging. As Dr. John Ratey says in one of my favorite books, *Spark: The Revolutionary New Science of Exercise and the Brain*: "Growing older is unavoidable, but falling apart is not."[4]

So how do we do this? How do we thwart Mother Nature as she marches us away from that strong and independent life we desire? In this book, I'll challenge many of the beliefs you hold regarding aging and your own wellness, and I'll show you strategies that allow you to age *your way* while building your lasting fitness.

EXERCISE

Write down ten issues you believe are contributing to your aging process (aside from the calendar). These could be physical (a chronic illness such as diabetes or heart disease), a family history of a certain disease, a long list of medications, bad eating habits, too much sitting, or not enough social or family support. Next to each issue, write down whether you believe this reason is something within your control.

_____

_____

_____

_____

_____

_____

_____

_____

_____

_____

TAKE CONTROL OF YOUR HEALTH

Who will take care of you when your health begins to fail in your seventies, eighties, or nineties? Will your family be able to support you? Will you have saved enough money or purchased adequate insurance? Will dependence on Social Security and Medicare let you age in comfort and safety? These are serious questions to consider, and as we saw above, ones that Americans are not completely prepared to address.

The population is aging, and the burden for families and the country are monumental. Consider the following statistics:

- American women are projected to live until age eighty-one, while men are projected to live until seventy-six.[5]

- By the year 2030, one in every five Americans—about 72 million people—will be an older adult.[6]

- Chronic diseases are the leading causes of death for older adults: heart disease and cancer, followed by stroke, chronic lower respiratory diseases, Alzheimer's disease, and diabetes.[7]

- Approximately 92 percent of older adults have at least one chronic disease, and 77 percent have two or more.[8]

- The cost of providing healthcare for one person aged sixty-five or older is three to five times higher than the cost for someone younger than sixty-five.[9]

- Today, more than two-thirds of all healthcare costs are for treating chronic illnesses.[10]

- Only 1 percent of health dollars are spent on preventive efforts to improve overall health.[11]

Chronic diseases lead to the loss of ability to perform everyday activities such as shopping, housekeeping, bathing, dressing, money management, and meal preparation. Older adults can become isolated, lonely, and depressed. Most Americans want to age in place, or live in their homes for as long as possible. To achieve this, they often require assistance.

A couple of years ago, I met a gentleman at a networking event who manages an in-home care company. I was surprised when he told me how difficult it is to keep good help because there is so much competition in the field now. The need for competent caregivers is growing significantly, and workers are easily lured from company to company. I've worked with clients who depend on caregivers, so when those caregivers change, the transition can be difficult and costly. The national average hourly fee for a home aide is $18 per hour with different state averages ranging from $15-25 if hired through an agency.[12]

Other clients of mine are lucky enough to have families help care for them. In fact, nationwide, approximately 43.5 million adult family caregivers are taking care of an older relative.[13] One of my sisters and I had been the primary caregivers for our mother in her later years, and I'm well aware of the mental stress and time commitment these tasks can exact.

We all want to live out our years in a fashion of our own choosing. But the truth is that 76 percent of us who want to die in our own homes will not be able to do that, according to my friend, Helen Justice, a geriatric care manager.

What opportunities do you have in your life for wellness? Are you passing them by? Clearly, the time to take charge of your health and wellness is now.

EXERCISE

Make a list of at least five exercise or healthy eating opportunities available to you that you are not taking advantage of. Are there free or low-cost exercise classes at the local senior center or park? Do you pass on that after-dinner walk with your spouse? Is there a farmer's market in your community with fresh, local produce? Are there cooking programs you could watch to pick up new recipe ideas? Start looking for possibilities and stop ignoring the ones already at your door.

_____

_____

_____

_____

_____

_____

GENETICS LOADS THE GUN; LIFESTYLE AND ENVIRONMENT PULL THE TRIGGER

Do you believe you're predisposed to a certain disease—your mother had it, your brother has it—so why bother modifying your diet or activity level? Should you just give up and let Mother Nature have her way?

When I started studying senior fitness, I was heartened to learn that most experts believe the chronic diseases we associate with aging are not actually a result of increasing years. I've learned that lifestyle is, in most cases, more important than the calendar. That's what I've taught my clients. I like to challenge them with this statement: They're not having problems walking because they're getting old; rather, they're getting old because they're not walking much any more.

So when I came across some statistics lately, they surprised me. According to the Center for Secure Retirement, 65 percent of Baby Boomers think their health is mostly determined by genes.

Less than half believe food and exercise are the key to wellness.[14] These folks will definitely shrug off the self-leadership role for their health. And some vocal people encourage them to. DJs at a radio station I listen to are quick to pick up the latest headlines about Alzheimer's or cancer and tell listeners, "See, it doesn't matter what you do. It's all up to your genes."

But this just isn't true. Even for those two deadly and feared diseases, lifestyle and environment can be a larger factor than your family tree.

In fact, we can probably all come up with exceptions to the "genes rule your destiny" myth. My mother had high blood pressure most of her life; mine has been well under control for as long as I can remember. My dad had cancer, and so far I'm clear on that one. But I know I carry that predisposition, and I've taken steps to up my chances for a healthy life. Of course, there are no guarantees.

But please take heed of these words from nationally renowned health and fitness expert Jonathan Ross: "The current thinking is that for most major degenerative diseases, genetics plays no greater role than 10% to 20%." Ross explains that while Alzheimer's rates are climbing rapidly as the population skews older (advancing age is the greatest risk factor for the disease), "only about 10% of cases carry the defective genes for the disease, and only half of those who carry the genes ever develop it. Most Alzheimer's cases are caused by cumulative brain damage that occurs during life." Disability and disease are not inevitable, despite your genes. As Ross goes on to conclude, "You've heard the saying about cars: 'It's not the years, it's the mileage.' The same is true for our bodies. Treat them rough and they wear out. Treat them well and they last longer while performing better."[15]

What do your genes say about your possibility of disease? When you visit a doctor for the first time, you always fill out a form about the illnesses your mother or father have. That's because they increase your risk for certain conditions, so healthcare professionals need to know what to watch for. But in most cases, they do not dictate your future. Can you take control of your wellness destiny and improve your chances for healthy aging?

EXERCISE

Compile a list of diseases that run in your family. Look closely at your parents and siblings. Put a checkmark next to conditions you believe you will inherit, ones you can "do nothing about." I'll have you do this exercise again at the end of the book to see whether you've changed your mind.

_____

_____

_____

THROW OUT ALL THOSE LABELS

Close your eyes and visualize a man or woman at eighty. What do you see? Is it an old person hunched over a walker, with shuffling feet as he or she moves slowly across the room? Or is it a vibrant, fit individual like Ernestine Shepherd, the gorgeous eighty-plus-year-old who holds the Guinness World Record as the world's oldest competitive female bodybuilder? Whatever you see, be careful—you're growing into that image.

Like many conditions in life, "aging" and "growing older" are just labels that become stereotypes. We can embrace them and let them control our lives, or we can ignore them. As I shared in the introduction, I had an experience with labels many years ago that sealed my belief in how detrimental they can be. At forty-two, I began experiencing double vision. This condition got so bad that I kept an eye patch in my car at all times. My kids, who were eight and twelve at the time, joked about me being a pirate. But the condition continued, and later I had problems with other facial muscles and started feeling weakness in my arms and legs.

I was eventually diagnosed with an incurable autoimmune disease called myasthenia gravis (Latin for "grave muscle weakness").

Uncertain of my future, I attended local support groups. And it was at those meetings, surrounded by sad people in neck braces and wheelchairs, that I decided to throw off the label. My future was not going to be looking like those people. With my doctor and husband, I chose a course of treatment that gave me the best chances for success, and I moved forward with my life.

At this point, I still have the disease. I can't donate blood, and I take immunosuppressants every day. But the myasthenia is so well controlled that my family forgets I have it and nobody who meets me would guess I have a muscle weakness disease. I've gone on to forge a career in fitness. I continue to strive for my 10,000 steps per day or 150 minutes of cardiovascular exercise per week and twice-weekly workouts at the gym. I even had fun reversing roles with my doctor recently by giving her exercise advice (quick tips for arms toning).

What labels are you embracing? Are they medical ("I'm diabetic") or related to your age ("I'm an old grandma")? Challenge yourself to throw off these beliefs, because that's all they are. Ernestine Shepherd sums it up, "Age is nothing but a number." I believe she's encouraging us all not to be limited by the calendar or the idea of "being old."

Another woman who smashes the paradigm of what our culture has taught us as the "standard after the age of fifty" is Dr. Christine Northrup, author of *Goddesses Never Age*.[16] Dr. Northrup maintains that what we call "aging" is chronic deterioration that begins in our twenties "when you start sitting all day," and gets worse as you age. She goes on to say this deterioration is not inevitable, and we all have the power to change that experience, "no matter what 'runs in your family' or what you've been told." She challenges us to write a new script, follow a new path. "It all starts with your beliefs. And the behavior that follows."[17]

EXERCISE

What labels and ageism beliefs are limiting your healthy, independent future? Here are a few examples I've heard: "I'm too old to do that," "I'm slowing down now," "Of course I have arthritis," "Growing old is a bitch." You may have to think hard about these ideas; they may not be obvious. They could be statements or observations from your childhood, comments from friends or family, or simply stereotypes you've picked up from our culture. Write down at least five beliefs you've internalized; the way to change them is first to acknowledge, then challenge them with the strategies I'll empower you with in this book.

_____

_____

_____

_____

_____

_____

SUMMARY

You've made it this far in life, so you're doing something right. Congratulations for that. But the remaining years can be challenging if you don't take control. In fact, the aging Baby Boomer population has been dubbed the "silver tsunami." We're a huge cohort of the population, and while we're living longer than our parents, we're not as healthy as they were at our age. Many experts fear our sheer numbers will overwhelm the healthcare system, and the statistics are pointing in that direction.

We want to live a long life, but the quality of those years is of paramount importance. Will you have the money and health to live out your life as you desire? None of us wants to become a burden to our families, and we want to stay independent for as long as possible.

But many of us are simply not making the choices that will bring that future to fruition. Fortunately, there is good news if we embrace healthy lifestyle changes: the World Health Organization predicts that with appropriate lifestyle changes, we can prevent at least 80 percent of all heart disease, stroke, and type 2 diabetes cases, and over 40 percent of cancer.[18]

So stop telling yourself "It runs in my genes," "I'm too old," or "I'm too weak to do that." Your mindset is critical for your enduring fitness. Ignore the calendar and turn back the hands of time with a commitment to your own wellness. Realize that it's actually cheaper and takes less effort to eat well and engage in physical activity than it is to be sick, on medications, in the hospital, or in a skilled nursing facility. With conscious and careful effort, it is possible to thwart Mother Nature. My clients have shown me this is true, and science has proven it as well!

CHAPTER 2

FINDING YOUR BIG "WHY"

"Once something is a passion, the motivation is there."

— Michael Schumacher

In the first chapter, you realized it's time to take control of your own health. Nobody else will do that. You now understand you *can* age your way, because in most cases, the lifestyle choices you make are more important than genetics. And remember, it's not that you can't get around any more because you're growing old; it's that you're growing old because you're not moving around any more!

As my clients say, "Do you want to take a stand, or do you want to let Mother Nature take her course?" I say you have to take a stand because that "course" is not a kind one, not a strong and self-sufficient one. It's not the road to your lasting fitness.

In this chapter, I'll help you find your true motivation or passion for the behavior changes that will keep you healthy and independent for years to come. You'll pinpoint that internal desire to pull you through the challenges that come up when life happens. Also helping you sustain lifestyle changes is discovering the joy of movement, in the moment, not four months from now when you see your doctor again. And finally, we'll look at risk-taking—a fear that often stops us from engaging in new behaviors—and ways to approach it safely.

OTHERS ARE ALWAYS NAGGING YOU

Just why are you embarking on this wellness journey? Is it because your doctor says you won't live long if you don't change your eating habits? Are you tired of your spouse arguing with you about sitting too much? Dozens of reasons can be found to pick up a phone and call a dietitian or personal trainer, or to join a weight-loss group or gym.

I've discovered over the years that the most successful clients are not the ones who contact me because their doctor referred them. In fact, many times these individuals decide they can't afford my services, even though they know they need them. Other people reach out to me because they decided *on their own* they have to change. Whether it's because they don't want to end up in a wheelchair, or they don't want the health complications of their parents with diabetes, they have their own reasons. And you'll need your reasons also to support yourself through months of change.

Scare tactics, while helpful for some, are generally not powerful motivators for change. In fact, they're what we call *extrinsic motivators*—incentives that come from outside sources.[1] They are often a good way to kick-start a new behavior change, but not a good motivation to continue with that change over the long haul. Personal trainer Jillian Michaels sums it up: "You can look for external sources of motivation and that can catalyze a change, but it won't sustain one. It has to be an internal desire." Michaels is reinforcing that an external motivation isn't enough to keep you going; you have to find a deeper goal.

The more powerful reason is an *intrinsic motivator*. It results when a person does physical activity for the inherent pleasure and experience that comes from the engagement itself.[2] Losing weight is intrinsically important if it leads to a sense of accomplishment or self-confidence, along with positive attitudes and emotions such as happiness, freedom, and relaxation. People who are intrinsically motivated will persist with a behavior change, even when faced with barriers.

My client Frank is perhaps the best example I've ever met of an intrinsically motivated person. He found me early in my fitness career a short time after he'd suffered a heart attack. He'd gained lots of weight over the years and become very sedentary. Even though he had a job that took him outdoors often, he rarely did fieldwork because he just couldn't walk the distances. Frank knew he had to change; his lifestyle was literally killing him. We worked for more than a year, through diet setbacks and injuries, until he lost the weight and regained his joy of life.

Frank's intrinsic motivation—the "carrot" that kept him going despite tough times in his fitness journey—was hiking. The more weight he lost, the farther he would walk, the higher he could go, and the more beauty in nature he could enjoy. Because he truly loved moving, his health journey became a self-perpetuating cycle. The better he ate, the more he could move. The more he moved, the more weight came off!

Frank found his big *why* and fully embraced it!

THE ONE BIG QUESTION YOU NEED TO ANSWER

"Why?" It's that simple: Why do you want to ___? It doesn't matter whether you desire to lose weight, get stronger, or find more energy. The key to your success will be to answer this question honestly: "Why do I want to ___?" You'll have to dig deep because it may not be obvious at first.

Why do you want to invest in going down the road of changing lifelong habits—be it eating or physical activity? Why do you want to invest the time (we're talking months initially, then maintaining new lifestyle changes *forever*)? What about the money it might cost? And the effort—getting off the sofa and moving when you'd rather keep sitting; pushing away from the table while there's still food left on your plate; spending extra time at the grocery store reading food labels.

We're not talking about a short-term goal that will lose its relevance once the special event has passed (cruise, wedding, or next doctor appointment).

Changing lifestyle behaviors takes a lot of effort! There's no way around it.

You know it's important. You know you need to make these changes. But when times get tough (and they will), it's critical to be able to call upon your true motivation to stay in the game.

For me, getting in shape and staying healthy means being around as long as possible to enjoy my family, especially the beautiful grandchildren. For one of my clients, it means staying out of a wheelchair. For Frank, it meant getting back to hiking, the hobby he loved but had given up as his health declined.

Can you find your big "why"? The answer to this question will be critical as you start your wellness journey and for months to come.

EXERCISE

Here's an example of one way to discover what really motivates you (as taught to me by one of my mentors, Jacqui Dobens):

Sit down at a table with someone you trust. For our example, I'll call this person Maggie. Be sure Maggie has a blank piece of paper and a pen or pencil; she'll need to record your responses.

Maggie: What is your goal?

You: To learn to eat better and lose thirty pounds.

Maggie: Why do you want to do this?

You: Because I want to improve control of my diabetes.

Maggie: Why do you want to have better control of your diabetes?

You: Because I want to get off my diabetes medications.

Maggie: Why do you want to get off your medications?

You: Because my medications have nasty side-effects and taking them means my blood sugar is too high.

Maggie: Why does it matter what your blood sugar numbers are?

You: Because I know that if I don't control my diabetes, I could lose my eyesight like my brother did, or die early from kidney disease like my father did.

Maggie: Why does that matter to you?

You: Because I want to enjoy a quality life with my kids as long as possible.

Now sit down and do this exercise with somebody who can ask you questions without judging.

And there you have it! You don't just want to improve your eating habits and lose thirty pounds because your doctor said you have to or because you're getting ready for your twenty-fifth high school reunion. You have a deeper motivation.

So when the chocolate cake looks tempting or you're feeling lazy, remember your true "why." Bring it back in full color. This motivation is what will help pull you through the ups and downs on the way to achieving your goals.

WHAT'S YOUR EXERCISE ECSTASY?

Why don't people exercise? By now, we all know it's good for us—our bodies and our minds. Yet 80 percent of Americans, including Baby Boomers and seniors, don't meet their physical activity recommendations.

How then, do you motivate yourself, or your loved ones, to move? Believe me, we personal trainers have been wrestling with that question for years!

One answer: Concentrate on the feeling! How do you *feel* during and after exercise? What's the immediate reward, not the long-term health benefits? Once you identify these positive emotions, you have a better chance of continuing with the activity.

Here are a few tips to get you in touch with your exercise ecstasy:

1. Stretch. Many of my clients love this activity—they tell me, "It just feels good!" Slowly easing into a stretch while breathing deeply, especially after exercise, creates a feeling of relaxation and eases tension. Many times, I hear my clients say, "I needed that!" after a tough day.

2. Focus on the feeling. I recently asked participants in one of my exercise classes to come up with some words describing how the activities made them feel. One of the best descrip-

tors I heard was "energized." It may sound counterintuitive—to feel more lively *after* exercising—but it's common to have more get-up-and-go following physical activity. I think we can all agree: Anything that gives us more energy as we age is definitely a plus!

3. Build confidence. Other words I hear often include "confident" or "accomplished." Again, this is especially important for older adults who can't visualize themselves lifting weights or riding a bicycle. Once they see they can do these activities successfully, they're more likely to try again.

4. Find your passion, an activity that brings you sheer joy! In the past, for me, this was bicycle riding. I love the feel of the wind through my hair, the sun on my face, and the green smells you miss while sitting in a car. More recently, the activity that gives me joy is silly dancing to fun songs with my grandkids or while doing chores. Music that moves me just brings a smile to my face. Which activity lights up your day?

5. Join others. Let's face it: We're social animals. While some people enjoy solitary activities, many love exercising with others to share success and create a sense of community. So find a senior exercise class at your local YMCA, learn ballroom dancing, or pick up a class schedule at your local junior college. Opportunities abound to be part of a "team" that warms your heart!

So, instead of forcing yourself to head out on that morning walk because it'll add years to your life, focus on more immediate feelings and identify the emotions related to physical activity that bring you joy. Then you'll be more likely to continue exercising, and the healthful benefits (of which there are dozens) will follow!

Can you find joy in movement? Challenge yourself to concentrate on the euphoria of the moment, not the health benefit that will occur down the road.

EXERCISE

List three activities you're willing to do on a consistent basis. These must be activities you enjoy performing; think outside the box if you must. Do you take pleasure in dancing, gardening (yes, it's considered moderate exercise), bicycling, swimming or water aerobics, tennis, or brisk walking after a meal or to watch the sun rise or set? Next to each activity, describe the "feeling" you get when you engage in the movement. We're looking for positive feelings, ones that will keep you going back to do that type of recreation.

_____

_____

_____

_____

_____

_____

_____

MORE TIPS BEFORE YOU START

Are you truly ready to make a commitment to change? Are you embarking on these lifestyle changes for *you*?

My very first client was Melissa, a teenage athlete. She got plenty of exercise, with five three-hour practices per week in her competitive sport. But Melissa was starting to have some health concerns possibly related to being overweight. Melissa's mother hired me because she wanted to find out why such an active teenager continued to gain weight.

I worked with my client for less than a month. I don't believe she was motivated to make the eating changes I recommended; they just weren't that important to her. Although she *said* she wanted to lose weight and learn to eat better, she really didn't feel it was a problem. She didn't follow my recommendations and didn't lose weight.

To me, Melissa epitomized a client reacting completely to an extrinsic factor. She had not yet internalized her need for behavior change. The "carrot" at the end of her journey just wasn't that important compared to eating with her fellow students during and after school.

EXERCISE

Take a good look at what's going on in your life. Write down a list of all the benefits you foresee in making your lifestyle change, along with an opposing list of the costs. Consider time, effort, money, and the fact that you'll be putting yourself out there for social ridicule or commendation. Do the benefits outweigh the costs?

_____

_____

_____

_____

AND FINALLY, DON'T BE AFRAID TO TAKE A RISK

How many times have you *not* started something because it *might not* turn out the way you want? You wish to begin a walking program, but your legs might hurt…. If you plant a garden for fresh veggies, the seedlings might die…. What if you don't find the time to ride that new bicycle you're thinking of buying?

Why bother?

Because *the things you're afraid of might never happen!* And what's the worst if they do? We know for sure what will happen if you don't take that risk—to quote ice hockey great Wayne Gretzky, "You miss 100% of the shots you don't take!"

Sometimes, you just have to look at the risk, take the necessary precautions, and jump in!

As an example, on a Sunday afternoon one winter, I needed to get away from my office. I only had 5,800 of my 10,000-step goal on my FitBit, and I had spent way too much time sitting. My favorite exercise is walking on our community "meadow" area. But it was cloudy and cold, and it had been drizzling. My phone was forecasting rain for another two hours.

If I stepped out for my thirty-minute walk, I might get wet and muddy! That has stopped me in the past.

But I was planning to bake chocolate chip cookies after dinner (my dreary weather indulgence), so I knew I had to burn off some calories ahead of time. So I put on a scarf, sweatshirt, and light windbreaker. I laced up a pair of hiking boots I didn't mind getting muddy, grabbed an umbrella, and walked out the door.

And it started raining…of course!

But I continued; the rain became a drizzle and stopped after ten minutes. By the time I got home, the scarf was off, the umbrella was useless, and both jackets were completely unzipped. And I was successful—my FitBit registered 9,903 steps!

The moral: Stop avoiding an important activity because you're afraid something might not go right!

Here are a few steps to consider before taking a risk:[3]

1. Increase your risk tolerance. Take risks in small doses to increase your self-confidence.

2. Stop underestimating yourself! You have many talents and abilities, so gather them up for self-confidence.

3. Consider the risks of settling. What are the consequences of not taking the risk?

4. Remember that risk is relative. Everybody has his or her own tolerance for risk, so don't compare yourself to others; find the right balance of risk-taking and routine-living to keep you moving forward.

5. Be realistic about what could go wrong. Keep consequences in perspective and prepare for them as best as possible.

6. Let go of what others think. (No additional info needed here!)

7. Picture everything going well. Athletes and speakers have mastered the skill of visualization; use positive thinking in seeing the results you desire.

SUMMARY

It is critical for your long-term success that you identify your internal motivation for getting fit and healthy. This true "why" is the only thing that will pull you through life's ups and downs as you work to change eating and physical activity habits. These new lifestyle choices have to last forever if you want to achieve your true wellness success and remain strong and independent. Make sure you took sufficient time to work through the exercise in this chapter to dig deep for your motivation.

Most people who start an exercise program don't continue it. It's just not fun. So we have to start focusing more on the positive feelings of activity during or right after we move. Don't rely on the long-term goal of losing weight or lowering blood sugar to keep you engaged in a new habit (which is uncomfortable and difficult for your brain to sustain). I can't get my husband to walk around the neighborhood with me because he doesn't enjoy it. However, he will attend yoga classes with me. He's found a joy in the stretches and the increased flexibility he feels immediately.

Find your own exercise joy!

Take stock of the pros and cons of your proposed behavioral change. Be honest and look at the time, money, and effort it will require. The positives have to outnumber the negatives, or you're just spinning your wheels. And don't be afraid to take a risk; you just might be surprised by the results. Take the necessary cautions and then jump right in. To end this chapter with another sports-related quote: "Just do it!"

CHAPTER 3

BUILDING THE GROUND-WORK FOR YOUR SUCCESS

"Motivation is what gets you started.
Habit is what keeps you going."

— Jim Ryun

You've decided to take control of your health—to age your way. And you've identified your reason to stay as healthy and independent as possible. Whether it's playing with your grandchildren, getting off all your medications, or saving money by living at home as long as possible, you now know your true "why."

Now it's time to lay the groundwork for your enduring fitness. Like everything worth doing, improving your wellness and strength takes constant effort and commitment. But while you're moving full blast in the right direction, life will always happen, throwing you off your course.

So in this chapter, I'll help you decide where you want to go with your wellness, give you encouragement to support your journey, and help you prepare for any obstacles you'll encounter.

ARE YOU JUST CHASING SQUIRRELS?

I often hear the following advice at business meetings: Don't go around chasing squirrels. In other words, keep the goal in mind and don't get sidetracked. This is true whether you're working on business intentions or personal ones. Have you written down your health or fitness goals—where you need to be in one week or one year to stay healthy and lead the life you want?

It's important to identify where you want to go, and then to break it down into workable chunks. The best way to do this is to come up with SMART goals. SMART is an acronym that stands for *specific, measurable, achievable, relevant,* and *time-bound.*

After you successfully reach a goal, reevaluate where you are and develop new SMART goals. Keep making small behavior changes—these reinforce self-efficacy: your belief in your ability to succeed in specific situations or to accomplish a task. And keep it simple!

I'll use the example of my client Frank to show you how this works. As I've already mentioned, Frank called me a few months after his heart attack. He was obese and had high blood pressure. He led a sedentary lifestyle with eating habits he knew were destroying his health. He wanted to lose seventy-five pounds, gain more muscle, and get off his blood pressure medication.

Because losing so much weight looked overwhelming, we broke his desire down to weekly goals. And we focused on tasks he could reasonably complete in a given timeframe, *not* weight-loss goals. For example, a weekly goal early in his program was to increase steps by an average of 500/day. This goal was specific, measurable, achievable, relevant, and tied to a timeframe. We gradually increased the number of steps in his goal, adding more targets like increasing the number of flights of stairs climbed.

All of these goals were completely within his control. Just walking the desired number of steps per day accomplished a goal and built his self-confidence. By focusing on *process* goals (something you can do), not *product* goals (something that is achieved, like "lose weight" or "get more healthy"), Frank continued to improve his health, eventually cutting his blood pressure medication in half and losing ninety pounds over eighteen months.

Have you looked seriously at your wellness goals? Have you taken time to break them down into bite-sized chunks? It's time to commit these to writing.

EXERCISE:

1. What are your long-term goals—those you want to achieve over the next 6-12 months? These could be tied in to your big "why," or maybe help get you to your "why." For example, you could want to: lose weight, decrease dependence on medications, improve balance, and play on the floor with your grandchildren.

2. Next, number your goals (if you have more than one) in order of priority, with number one being the most important.

3. Record your relevant baseline information, for example, the number of steps or minutes per day you're walking, the amount of medication you're taking, your health numbers (blood pressure, blood sugar/glucose or A1C, blood lipids—total cholesterol, low-density lipoprotein (LDL), high-density lipoprotein (HDL)). These values are important for tracking progress.

4. Now think about or investigate what it might take to reach your first goal—broken into short-term targets. If you need help, ask your healthcare professional.

5. Finally, pick out one goal you can write as a SMART goal. Make it a weekly goal.

Let's take the example of my client, Martha, who was overweight and took medications for type 2 diabetes. We decided to start by improving her eating habits, and her first weekly goal was to decrease her soda intake from two 20-oz. servings per day to one.

*   *Specific* (decrease from two to one)
*   *Measurable* (track soda intake)
*   *Achievable* (we're not asking her to change her entire eating pattern)
*   *Relevant* (sodas contribute lots of calories and sugar to the diet—important for a gal with type 2 diabetes who carries extra weight)
*   *Time-bound* (one week timeframe)

On the lines below, list out your pertinent health data. Then write out one SMART goal, showing how it's specific, measurable, achievable, relevant, and time-bound.

_____

_____

_____

_____

_____

_____

_____

_____

IT TAKES A COMMUNITY

Now that you know where to go, are you making that journey alone, or with the help of others? Some people prefer not to draw attention to themselves; others want to avoid meddling questions when they start changing their eating and activity habits. But when it comes to fitness, it's best to invite others to support your efforts.

One of my clients, Barbara, hired me for just four sessions to help her put into place the heart-healthy diet recommendations she'd received in a class at Loma Linda University Medical Center. In addition to our weekly sessions, she attended a Weight Watchers program. The ladies in these meetings shared a common weight-loss journey. Since Barbara lived alone and had no family close by, her Weight Watchers "friends" cheered her successes and helped each other through rough eating situations.

One of the best predictors of success in a behavior-change program is support.[1] That support can take the form of family members, friends, social media groups, gym members, etc. Buddies can support you in many ways:

- They help keep you motivated and accountable. For example, you'll be much more likely to take that morning walk if you know someone is counting on you.

- Researchers know that people tend to exhibit health behaviors similar to those around them. You can increase your level of self-control or commitment when you surround yourself with other like-minded individuals. On the flip side, your efforts can crash if others perform less than optimal health behaviors.

- Buddies can help you through challenging situations, listening without judgment and offering encouragement.

- Spouses are especially influential in positive health behavior change. And studies have shown that change is more successful if both partners are moving away from unhealthy behaviors together.

- You can formalize your "partnership" with a life coach, personal trainer, or registered dietitian. These health professionals will educate you and keep you accountable.

Some people may be jealous or uncomfortable with your fitness or eating changes. They may consciously or unconsciously sabotage your efforts. If you feel this is happening, talk with the saboteur, ask whether he or she can identify what might be the problem, and gently ask for his or her support. Most people will correct their behaviors once they're aware of them.

What does your support system look like? Do you even have one? Take a serious look at those who might be able to encourage you as you begin to make important lifestyle changes.

EXERCISE

Brainstorm ten ways to build a supportive community for your behavior-change journey. List specific people (your spouse, your siblings, your children, or your coworkers). Think about where you interact with people who could help you—a senior center, bowling alley, crafts or card club, church—any place you can enlist the support of people who would like to see you be successful in building and maintaining your fitness.

Now list the specific support you need to ask for from each person. Here are some examples:

- To a spouse: Will you congratulate me when I start using smaller plates or eating a salad at each dinner?

- To a coworker: Will you join me every morning break for a fifteen-minute walk?

- To a sibling: It would help if somebody checked in with me on my exercise program once a week; could you do that?

Then, write in a date or time when you will talk with that person, and check off this information when you've completed it.

_____

_____

_____

_____

_____

STACK THE ODDS IN YOUR FAVOR, AND OTHER STRATEGIES

You've identified a specific behavior you wish to change, and you've enlisted friends and family for support, but how are you going to make it a habit? How are you going to find the time or remember to exercise, stand up more often, eat a healthy snack, or drink more water?

As a personal trainer, I know the importance of working out on a regular basis, and I need to keep my muscles in pretty good shape. But sometimes it's just hard to get myself out of the house and into the gym. I've learned I'm much more likely to enter the gym if I'm already driving around, so I look at my calendar each week and write in days/times when I work with a client, and then go to the gym afterwards. I'm stacking that behavior (gym) on top of a relevant behavior I'm already doing (meeting clients). That way I'm much more successful at meeting my own workout goals.

Stacking is an easy way to establish a new habit.[2] You do it by linking the new behavior to an existing one. The theory is that your brain is already wired to do certain tasks every day. If you stack a new behavior onto a well-established routine, you're much more likely to accomplish it.

The keys to successful stacking include:

- Start by making a list of your existing routines, for example, brushing your teeth in the morning and evening, making coffee each day, or checking your email.

- Next, be specific and look for a stack that makes sense. For example, *I'll drink 8 ounces of water every time I check my email*, or *I'll take a fifteen-minute walk after doing the dishes*.

- Don't overwhelm yourself with too many behaviors.

EXERCISE

List five behaviors you already do every day, such as brushing your teeth, drinking coffee, sitting down to watch TV at night, or checking social media every morning. Next, team one of them with a behavior change you intend to change this week.

1. _____

2. _____

3. _____

4. _____

5. _____

A recent article looks at the science of habit formation. The author first explains habits in terms of what goes on in the brain.[3] While it's fairly complex, the bottom line is that the part of the brain where an old, engrained habit resides *always* wins over the area trying to form the new behavior. And because more than 40 percent of our daily behaviors are done habitually, it takes a consistent plan to make lasting changes.

The author recommends looking at the cue-behavior-reward loop. The cue is an environmental or internal trigger that causes us to learn a behavior. The behavior is the actual routine or "habit." The reward or incentive is what promotes some kind of pleasure to make a behavior recur.

Because of the way our brains are wired, the article urges readers to change the *behavior*, not the cue or reward. For example, let's say you watch your grandchildren one night every week. Each time they come over, you go out for ice cream—your rational side knows it's not particularly healthy for anybody, but your emotional side knows it'll taste great and make the little ones happy!

Instead of changing the cue (you love having the kids come over) or the reward (you all want to feel good), change the behavior. Find another activity. Maybe you can make "homemade" popcorn, or go outside and play with bubbles. You still have the cue/grandchildren twice a week, and you still have a great feeling for everybody, but the new habit will be more healthful all around!

EXERCISE

Identify one cue-behavior-reward system you'd like to break. It could be an eating habit or a sedentary behavior. Then come up with two substitute behaviors or habits that will easily slip in between the other two parts of the formula.

LIFE HAPPENS!

Do you spend weeks working on healthful new behaviors, only to be totally derailed by life? Do you get discouraged, convinced you can never go on vacation or enjoy a meal out again?

When I work with clients, I always ask them the same question before a weekend: What obstacles might come up in the next few days that will throw your plans off? For Margaret, it was often dinner or card games with fellow Baby Boomers at their fifty-plus community. So we would put together a list of strategies to help her navigate eating situations, with different ideas depending on whether she was hosting the event or visiting somebody else's home.

For Bob, a fishing vacation in Alaska fell in the middle of our training time. Eating wasn't going to be a problem, but he was concerned about sitting all day on a boat and all night talking with the guys in the cabin. We put together a plan to incorporate walking and regular movement to keep his steps on par.

As I said above, "Life happens" and it's meant to be enjoyed! Luscious desserts are plentiful on a cruise, birthday celebrations occur, people gather around the kitchen snacking on chips and dip, or you just want to be lazy on your vacation.

Go ahead, indulge! To get back on track, you need to learn resilience—the ability to recover quickly from the surprises and detours of life. I always urge my clients not to try for perfection, but rather to follow their plans 80-90 percent of the time; for the other 10-20 percent, enjoy; then get back to your good habits as quickly as possible.

EXERCISE

Take out your calendar and look at events coming up in the next week that might put a detour in your fitness plans. Write out a specific strategy to counter these effects.

_____

_____

_____

_____

_____

Here are a few more helpful hints from the American Council on Exercise:[4]

1. At the beginning of your new behavioral journey, track your progress with self-monitoring. Try a program like SuperTracker[5] or MyFitnessPal.[6] You'll learn more about tracking behaviors

in upcoming chapters, but record your food and water intake, along with exercise, for a week and then see which behaviors you might want to modify. If you've already made a goal, see how well you've kept it.

2. Avoid negative self-talk. We are our worst enemies. The next time you find yourself saying, "This is too difficult," "I'm too lazy," or "I'm too big to exercise," stop and replace negativity with positive thoughts. Instead, congratulate yourself for any steps you've made toward your fitness goals, such as "I'm so proud of myself for drinking six glasses of water today," or "I'm awesome because I walked this morning!"

3. To increase your motivation, find a reward for completing a major goal. Celebrated successes will increase the likelihood of future accomplishments. Buy that fancy new kitchen utensil you've wanted, see a movie, or attend a concert.

4. Increase the potential for success by setting up an environment to support your efforts. For example, if you want to go to the gym in the morning, keep an extra pair of shorts and shoes in the car. Place healthful foods in front of those you wish to avoid.

MAKING TIME FOR ACTIVITY

Is this the biggest reason you don't exercise: You're too busy and just can't find the time? It's a complaint I frequently hear when speaking with potential clients; in fact, it's the number-one reason people give for not exercising.[7]

We all know we need more physical activity, but between jobs, social commitments, and caring for parents or grandchildren, we have difficulty fitting it into our days.

The truth is, you'll never "find" time for exercise. You have to "make" the time because life will always get in the way, casting off your best intentions right and left!

Here are five strategies to help you carve out precious minutes for physical activity:

1. **Put it on your calendar:** You "calendar" your meetings, manicures, and phone conferences, so why not give exercise the same consideration? Commit to a specific day and time, record the appointment in a spot you'll see on a regular basis, and schedule reminders as needed. As a result, you're much more likely to get to these activities.

2. **Exercise with a buddy:** Plan to be active with a friend or family member. As I've said before, you'll coax each other along, and neither of you will want to let the other down.

3. **You don't need a thirty-minute block of time:** Good news! You can break your physical activity into ten- or fifteen-minute increments. So no more excuses—if you're working, you have ten-minute breaks every day! Keep your tennies under your desk, and walk instead of sitting or eating. Then look for a few minutes in the morning or evening to eke out other mini-exercise breaks.

4. **Understand that any movement is better than none:** If you can't find time for the recommended 150 minutes per week, don't stress. Even a few minutes of exercise each day are beneficial.

5. **Track your activity every thirty minutes during one weekday and one weekend day.** I've used this strategy with a few clients to help them discover exercise possibilities. Don't make a big deal out of it—use whatever method works best

for you (paper and pencil, your phone, or a computer). The idea is to locate "down time." You'll be surprised how often you watch TV, chat on the phone, or catch up on Facebook. These pockets of time are golden when you're looking to get more movement into your day.

SUMMARY

In this chapter, we've spent a lot of time looking at various strategies to help you be successful on your wellness journey. First and foremost, you must identify your goals, both long-term (6-12 month) and short-term (2-3 month). Next, "chunk" these down into manageable weekly targets that become SMART goals—specific, measurable, achievable, relevant, and time-bound.

Track your progress at the end of each week; revise goals as needed. Learn to increase the possibility of maintaining a new behavior by stacking habits, celebrating your achievements, replacing negative self-talk with positive statements, and creating a supportive environment.

You can't make this journey on your own, so enlist others' help. Find like-minded people who can help you be accountable for your actions, boost your motivation, and offer encouragement. Avoid people whose negative health behaviors might rub off on you. And deal with those who might consciously or unconsciously sabotage your efforts. Try to find the reason for their undermining comments and ask for their support.

Don't sit around waiting for exercise time to fall into your lap (it's not going to happen). Use the strategies in this chapter (and the next) to make more movement in your life.

And finally, recognize that life happens—always! Don't expect perfection, but aim to follow your new habits 80-90 percent of the time. When you eat too much or move too little because of a vacation or special event, don't get down on yourself—just return to your goal behaviors as soon as possible. Remember, it takes weeks to develop a new habit, and you're trying to undo behaviors that have taken a lifetime to establish.

CHAPTER 4

MOVING—EVERY DAY!

"Be not afraid of going slowly; be afraid only of standing still."

— Ancient Chinese proverb

In the previous chapter, we set the foundation for your successful journey to lasting fitness. We made sure your eyes were focused on a goal, you had built-in support systems, you developed new habits, you looked for ways to prepare for obstacles, and you enlisted somebody to keep you accountable. In this chapter, we'll begin exploring the new science of movement, why movement is vitally important, and how to get more of it in your life.

WE'VE ENGINEERED MOVEMENT OUT OF OUR LIVES

Do you leave your vacuuming to a Roomba? Have you given up stair-climbing for the ease of an escalator? Is your office designed for maximum efficiency so you don't take any extra steps? If you answered "yes" to these questions, welcome to our modern life—where convenience is king and movement is dying!

I had a real eye-opening experience several years ago. My husband and I went to see the movie *WALL-E* with our grandchildren. It's a sweet story set in 2805, when a threat to humanity has caused Earthlings to flee the planet and take refuge on a starliner, leaving behind a lovable robot, WALL-E. Over the centuries, people grew lazy—with machines bringing them food whenever desired—and eventually, they became obese and unable to walk. This, my friends, is where we're headed unless we make some drastic changes.

In fact, a recent newspaper article confirmed my fears.[1] McDonald's and Uber-Eats are teaming up in my Southern California area to bring your favorite fast food right to your door. Now you have even less reason to walk to your car for that quick "dining out" experience!

Let me share a story about one of my clients, Robert. I'd known Robert and his family from several years back. It had been almost two decades since I'd seen them when his wife showed up for one of my workshops. Robert had gained forty pounds over the past fifteen years, so she was concerned for his health.

Although Robert's regular job involved walking outside, he was glued to a chair four hours a day working a second job. He had everything he needed at his fingertips, so getting up and walking around wasn't required often.

One topic I talk about with new clients is how much they move. Robert believed he walked enough at his main job. But when he checked the steps that his phone had been tracking for months, he was clocking a mere 3,000 steps daily!

Along with making major food changes, we put together a plan for Robert to increase his daily activity. He recently texted me with an update. Robert's now averaging 14,000 steps per day and has lost thirty-one pounds in twelve months. His advice: *You have to move. Every day!*

Robert is a typical example of what's happening in our country now. *Sedentary behavior, or sitting time, has become a public health problem.* We spend prolonged periods sitting or lying down—computer use, screen time, television watching, or commuting.

According to Dr. James A. Levine, director of the Mayo Clinic/Arizona State University Obesity Solutions and author of *Get Up: Why Your Chair Is Killing You and What You Can Do About It!*, we now sit for thirteen hours a day, sleep for eight, and move for three.[2] We no longer have physically-challenging jobs; the energy we expend on household tasks has dropped significantly, and we're addicted to our smartphones!

As you'll see below, it's imperative that we begin breaking up sitting time. How can you get more movement back into your life?

EXERCISE

In the lines below, write out ten activities you can include in your daily routine. I'm not talking about exercise, but rather movement that you've lost. Maybe you can fire your housekeeper or gardener. How about moving all your trash cans to one room so you have to get up more often? Or walking while you're on the phone? Or parking at the far end of the lot? What about using stairs instead of the escalator?

_____

_____

_____

_____

_____

IT'S THE NEW SMOKING—ARE YOU GUILTY?

You've given up your daily sodas (excellent!) and you stopped smoking (even better!). But are you unknowingly engaging in a behavior all the time that's even more unhealthy?

I worked with an eighty-one-year old client, Sam, who had been wheelchair-bound for two to three years. He was a diabetic, on insulin. He and his wife ate very few high-sugar foods, but occasionally splurged on chocolate chip cookies. Although his appetite wasn't very big, his blood sugar was often on the high side. I believe this was partially because he was so sedentary. His body's fuel supply (blood sugar or glucose) simply wasn't needed to support activity.

Along with diabetes, Sam was suffering from the new "sitting disease." One of the first studies to identify this problem was completed at the middle of the last century in London.[3] Researchers in England hypothesized that men in physically active jobs would have a lower incidence of coronary heart disease compared to those in less physically active jobs. To prove their hypothesis, they looked at medical and absence records of drivers and conductors on the London transport system of buses, trams, and trolleybuses in the 1950s.

They found the annual rate of heart disease for drivers, who spent their time sitting, was 2.7 per 1,000. But it was 1.9 per 1,000 for conductors, who moved about the vehicles collecting tickets. The investigators concluded that employees in positions requiring high physical activity had lower rates of coronary heart disease.

Dr. Levine has been a leader in the modern study of obesity and inactivity. He writes that our bodies are built for movement. Up until 100 years ago, our ancestors engaged in agricultural activities, sitting for only a few hours a day. But life has changed.

When you stop moving for an extended number of hours, it's like telling your body it's time to shut down and prepare for death. Dr. Levine's investigations show that when you've been sitting for a long period of time and then get up, a number of molecular reactions occur. For example, within ninety seconds of standing up, you start pushing blood sugar and fats out of the bloodstream and into the cells to be used for energy. All of these effects are started just by carrying your own bodyweight, and if done regularly, they can greatly decrease your risk of diabetes and obesity.

Other investigators have documented additional health risks of sitting. A 2015 issue of *Annuals of Internal Medicine* reviewed forty-seven studies and concluded that sedentary behavior is associated with increased risk of diabetes, heart disease, and cancer, and a higher risk of dying from all causes.[4] Other researchers add the risk of developing dementia, obesity, depression, and back pain to the list.

According to the World Health Organization, approximately 3.2 million deaths each year are attributable to insufficient physical activity.[5] In fact, Dr. Levine states, "For every hour you sit, two hours of life walk away."[6]

Are you guilty, then, of sabotaging your own health simply by the number of hours you sit per day? Even if you've made positive changes to your diet, get plenty of sleep, and manage your stress—the very act of not moving is making you sick!

YOU EXERCISE REGULARLY—BUT YOU'RE STILL UNHEALTHY

Have you finally figured out a way to fit a 45-60 minute walk into your day, but otherwise, you lead a sedentary lifestyle? That's a start, but don't feel too smug about the walking part because there's still a problem.

When I worked at a gym, I talked with many people who came in regularly. I noticed that most of the older folks spent their time on the treadmill; their minutes at the gym two or three times a week were the sum of their activity. They came week after week, but they never lost weight or seemed healthier.

For those gym-goers who became my clients, we took a different approach. We looked at life *outside* the gym and found ways to get them off their chairs as often as possible.

As it turns out, we now know that going to the gym a few days a week, or even walking an hour a day, won't undo the unhealthy effects of inactivity the rest of the day. People who get up frequently and move all day long actually use more energy and are healthier than those who sit and get their 30-60 minutes of exercise.

The new science of wellness tells us that even if we manage the recommended 150 minutes of exercise per week, that's not enough to stay healthy. In fact, prolonged sitting will actually negate the benefits of a concentrated bout of activity. That's right—six hours of reclining cancels out the fitness gains of a sixty-minute workout!

That's come as a surprise to many of us in the fitness field—one hour of physical activity will not overcome the negative effects of six to eight hours of continuous sitting. How can that be?

To understand, we have to look at the human body.

We burn calories in three ways. The first is basal metabolic rate (BMR), which is the minimum amount of energy our body needs to stay alive at rest. BMR accounts for 60 percent of the calories we expend. Second is the thermic effect of food, or the number of calories it takes to "process" our food. This amounts to about 10 percent of the calories we burn. And that leaves activity thermogenesis, which torches 30 percent of calories daily.

This last category holds the key to health.

It's all because of a concept called NEAT. Here's how it works. Activity thermogenesis has two components: what we think of as traditional exercise and what's called non-exercise activity thermogenesis (NEAT). NEAT is energy expended for everything we do that is not sleeping, eating, or intentional sports-like exercise. It ranges from calories burnt for walking to talking, gardening, standing, and toe tapping.[7]

NEAT is by far the largest portion of activity thermogenesis, and the component we can affect the most to benefit health.

Every movement requires energy and burns calories. (You burn 25 percent more calories simply by going from lying down to sitting in a chair and answering email.) What studies have shown is that people with obesity have a low-NEAT calorie burn. One research project revealed they sat 135 minutes more per day than lean volunteers. Clearly, the more you move, all day long, the more calories you burn and the more you promote positive physiological processes in your body.

How then, do we increase NEAT? Most people struggle to meet the recommendation of 150 minutes of exercise per week, so how do we get even more movement in our lives? While it sounds discouraging, think of it this way: 150 minutes a week is less than 2 percent of your waking hours. And that leaves lots of time for activity, with the key being frequent and consistent movement.

And the research is now clear: It is imperative to stand up and move more often! The American Diabetes Association (ADA) is the first organization I've seen to officially embrace this advice.[8] Its 2017 Standards of Care recommend, along with the 150 minutes of moderate-to-vigorous physical activity per week, "All adults, and particularly those with type 2 diabetes should decrease the amount of time spent in daily sedentary activity. Prolonged sitting should be interrupted every 30 minutes for blood glucose benefits...."

So the best way to improve health is:

- *150 minutes of moderate-to-vigorous physical activity per week* (not only recommended by the ADA, but also the Department of Health and Human Services, the American Heart Association, and the American Council on Exercise)

—PLUS—

- *light activity (about two minutes) to break up sedentary time every 30-60 minutes*

If you're having difficulty "finding" time for daily movement, here are five ideas to get you started:

1. **Become less efficient.** If you're still working, inform your boss that employees who are physically active throughout the workday are more productive. Then she won't mind when you begin to print to another office, use the upstairs restroom, or hold "walking" meetings.

2. **Embrace your work break time.** A full-time employee has at least sixty minutes of free time each day—a gift for movement! Get your buddies involved and stroll on a regular basis.

3. **Seek out the stairs instead of elevators and escalators.**

4. **Get creative with indoor walking.** Many malls now welcome walking visitors and indicate the distance per "lap"—in year-round, air-conditioned comfort.

5. **Move more throughout the day!** Play a guitar or piano, walk your dog, clean a room, carry groceries, and play with your kids or grandchildren. Or just pretend you're a child and

do the things we ask them not to do: fidget, tap your toes, stand on one foot and then the other when standing in lines, or dance—just don't stay still!

How can you add regular movement and activity into your life?

EXERCISE

List ten ways you can increase your NEAT. Think in terms of *movement or activity*, not exercise:

1. _____

2. _____

3. _____

4. _____

5. _____

6. _____

7. _____

8. _____

9. _____

10. _____

WHEN IGNORANCE ISN'T BLISS

Like many of my clients, do you think you spend a lot of time moving during the day? Are you sure, and just how do you know?

As I mentioned with Robert, who thought he walked enough because of his job, most people overestimate their physical activity.[9] As a result, they don't think they have to work at getting in more steps or movement. But in my experience, exactly the opposite is true!

One of the first things I ask my clients to do is to buy a pedometer or activity tracker to find out what their baseline activity level is. I have them record the steps over a week; then we review the information and begin setting goals: for example, increasing 200 steps each day.

Even clients who do not take normal, forceful steps can record their activity. We always find a way to make this happen, as with my octogenarian client, Dorothy, who has a neurological disease. Because of the effects this condition has on her legs, her short shuffling steps do not register when a pedometer is attached at her waist—the normal spot we'd put it. Even wearing a tracker on her arm did not accurately record steps. Our solution was to tie the pedometer onto her shoe with her shoestrings and multiply this number by two. Now each step is accounted for, and she can gradually increase her movement.

I have a FitBit, and I love it! Like many users, I'm rather addicted to having it give me information constantly. A few months ago, the black wristband fell apart—literally. The FitBit folks sent me a new one, but while I waited for it, I had no idea what my activity level was. This was a very uncomfortable feeling since I normally aim for 10,000 steps per day and have been known to walk up and down the hall before bedtime until I reach my goal. With no record of my steps, I had no idea how I was doing.

(Addendum: During the writing of this book, hip arthritis pain with walking became so bad I had to give up counting steps. Now I aim for 150 minutes per week on my stationary bicycle.)

While studies vary as to whether wearable fitness technology actually increases activity, it is an excellent way to establish baseline movement and track improvement.

I've worked with other clients who prefer to monitor the number of minutes they move (not steps), or the minutes between movement. These folks aim to get the 150 minutes of exercise weekly, along with getting up every hour or so to move. You can check your computer or smartphone to see whether you can set an alarm or reminder every 30-60 minutes. My daughter had a Garmin that shook her wrist and flashed when she hadn't gotten up after an hour. If technology is simply not your forte, you can always set an alarm in your kitchen to get you off the sofa every hour.

You can pick up a pedometer at a store like Target or WalMart for as low as $10.00. Do not buy anything too complicated—your main goal is to track steps daily. The more expensive activity trackers (FitBit, Garmin, MisFit) run from about $50-$250. The Apple Watch will cost over $350. All these devices do slightly different tracking, so check out the various models at a sporting goods store, and the Apple product at your Apple Store. Also check online for many product reviews and comparisons.

Is it time for you to start tracking, and increasing, your movement? Whether it's a simple pedometer, an Apple Watch, a FitBit, or other activity tracker, your body thanks you!

THREE NIGHTS IN THE HOSPITAL, A WEEK IN REHAB

Do you think that, because you're getting older, activity isn't that important any more? Think all this fuss about movement is just for young people?

You couldn't be more wrong!

The last time my mother entered a hospital, the doctor wanted to keep her for two to three nights after a fall. He told us that, upon discharge, she would have to go to a rehab center for *at least a week.* His reasoning was that the amount of time in bed would weaken her legs so much she'd have to relearn how to use her walker. We were shocked at how quickly she would lose her strength.

Then I saw a study that looked at inactivity in younger people, and it all made sense. In research conducted at the Institute of Aging and Chronic Disease, University of Liverpool, UK, twenty-eight participants (average age twenty-five) were asked to decrease their steps from 10,000 per day to 1,500.[10] In just two weeks, they started losing muscle mass, while increasing body fat. And their fitness levels dropped. These were healthy young people; it's no wonder inactivity hits older people so hard.

Can you afford *not* to pay attention to your activity level and continue ignoring ways to increase movement?

EXERCISE

List at least five activities that keep you on your bottom for extended periods of time. They could include computer time, Facebook time, phone time, working Sudoku or crossword puzzles, reading time, or television watching. Now brainstorm and write down five ways to get yourself up every 30-60 minutes. For example, stand and walk around during every commercial or at the start of every new TV show; do the same at the end of each chapter, or walk around while on the phone. Find something that will work for you. Use some of the stacking techniques you learned in Chapter 2 to connect movement with habits you already have.

Dr. Levine's goal is to decrease total sedentary time by two hours and fifteen minutes per day.

Sedentary Activities	Ways to Break Up Sedentariness
_____	_____
_____	_____
_____	_____
_____	_____
_____	_____
_____	_____
_____	_____

SUMMARY

We have become very efficient in our lives, with lots of labor-saving devices that have allowed us to become lazy. Sedentary time has increased significantly, with most of us spending more than half our waking hours sitting or lying down. In fact, TV-watching (highly correlated with sedentary time) is the number-one leisure activity of older adults.

As our daily movement has decreased, the connection with chronic diseases has risen: Sitting is associated with an increased risk of coronary heart disease, type 2 diabetes, some cancers, dementia, obesity, depression, back pain, and a higher risk of dying from all causes.

Our sitting behavior is killing us—for every hour you sit, you lose two hours of life.

And recent studies reveal the surprising news that you can exercise for an hour and still be unhealthy—if you're sedentary the rest of your day. This seems counterintuitive, but people who move (not "exercise") throughout their days are actually more healthy than those who sit most of the time and get up for a scheduled gym workout or walking time.

The way we can turn the tables in our favor is by increasing NEAT calories. NEAT refers to non-exercise activity thermogenesis, and it's everything we do that's not sleeping, digesting food and turning it into energy, or planned exercise.

We talked previously about taking a self-leadership role in your own wellness. Here is a perfect place to put that into practice by reviewing your own sedentary time and looking for ways to break it up. Engage in activities that move you—from fidgeting to fighting with your vacuum cleaner.

Aim for 10,000 steps per day or 150 minutes of moderate-to-vigorous physical activity per week, while standing for two minutes with light movement to exercise the large muscles in your legs every 30-60 minutes.

And don't forget to put in place reminders for activity and ways to monitor movement. Pedometers and activity trackers are great motivators to get up and walk and to increase movement with time.

CHAPTER 5

FOCUSING ON A PLANT-BASED DIET

"If beef is your idea of 'real food for real people,' you'd better live real close to a real good hospital."

— Neal Barnard, MD

By now, I hope you realize that while longevity begins with genes, the real key to healthy aging is lifestyle choices. Along with the proper mindset and support, movement throughout the day is critical for adding healthy years to your life. It's not just the thirty minutes of exercise you get five days per week; it's also the time you spend off your chair—walking, doing chores, climbing stairs—that could add years of quality living.

In this chapter, we'll explore the dietary connection for supporting a longer life.

LESSONS FROM THE BLUE ZONES

Just what are the secrets to living to 100? As we saw in Chapter

1, most Americans wish to live that long. In 2003, award-winning author and researcher Dan Buettner, in conjunction with *National Geographic* and funded in part by the National Institutes of Aging, set off to discover the answer.

His journey took him to places he refers to as the Blue Zones—regions where people outlive the rest of us by decades. These places include Japan; Costa Rica; Italy; Greece; and Loma Linda, California. Along with natural activity, reducing stress, and finding purpose and belonging in their lives, Buettner discovered the centenarians in these areas ate simple, home-prepared foods—primarily plant-based.[1]

Food for the eighty-, ninety- and one-hundred-year olds in the Blue Zones comes from their own gardens and orchards. These people depend heavily on beans (fava, black, soy, and lentils—excellent non-meat sources of protein), whole grains (containing fiber, antioxidants, potential anti-cancer agents, cholesterol reducers, and clot blockers, along with essential minerals), nuts, vegetables, and fruits.

However, most people in the Blue Zones are not strict vegetarians; they eat meat sparingly, a serving the size of a deck of cards, an average of five times per month. And that's the size of an adult deck of cards, not your grandkids' oversized deck of Fish cards. They eat no processed, "junk" or high-caloric density foods (foods that contain a high number of calories compared to the nutrition they contribute; think soda or candy).

A healthy plant-based diet includes foods with the opposite quality—high-*nutrient* density—and minimizes processed foods, fats, and animal products. These diets have been shown to be beneficial for:

• weight loss[2]

- decreasing the risk of diabetes[3]
- decreasing incidence and death from heart disease[4]
- lowering blood pressure[5]

A study published in 2017 provided support for decreasing meat intake. The researchers concluded an increase in red meat consumption increases the risk of dying from eight diseases, including cancer, heart disease, respiratory diseases, stroke, diabetes, infections, and kidney and liver disease.[6]

When I was working on my internship to become a personal trainer, I spent several weeks at the cardiac rehab program, Scripps Memorial Hospital in La Jolla, California. As a "student," I was invited to participate in all aspects of this multi-faceted program. In one key component, dietitians conducted nutrition and cooking classes focused on a vegetarian diet. Healthcare professionals in the program felt strongly that patients needed to find ways to get high-fat meat products out of their diets so they could better embrace their new heart-healthy lifestyle. The emphasis was on teaching patients to prepare tasty meatless foods they could easily substitute for their usual dietary fare (for example, we enjoyed a tofu "egg" salad).

These participants, having suffered a heart attack, were highly motivated to make healthy changes to their diets. What will it take for you to modify your eating habits? Hopefully, you won't wait until clogged arteries land you in the ER.

EXERCISE

Write down five reasons you need to change your diet. These could be medical conditions (obesity, high blood pressure, prediabetes) or personal (you want to save money by not dining out so often, you want to model healthy eating habits for your grandchildren).

_____

_____

_____

_____

_____

EAT LIKE YOU'RE ON A SUNNY VACATION

Need further incentive to spend more time in the produce aisle? Imagine eating a diet that reduces the risk of heart attacks, heart disease, and stroke by 30 percent[7], and also reduces the risk of type 2 diabetes and breast cancer. Just take your eating habits to sunny Italy or Greece.

Scientists have studied the dietary and lifestyle patterns in the Mediterranean region for more than fifty years. While the diet has long been associated with a lower risk of heart disease, dozens of well-designed studies have pointed to other exciting results. This lifestyle also supports healthy brain aging. For example, in one study of older adults, Mediterranean diet followers were more likely to have a protective association against brain atrophy.[8]

Incorporating principles of this lifestyle into your own is not difficult. Similar to eating habits in the Blue Zones, the plan emphasizes consuming primarily plant-based foods—fruits and vegetables, whole grains, legumes (dried peas and beans), seeds, nuts, and olive oil. It recommends eating low-fat cheese and yogurt as the main dairy products (these contribute calcium and vitamin D for strong bones, and help control blood pressure), and fish and poultry only occasionally (fish is high in omega-3 fatty acids, essential nutrients that our bodies cannot make; omega-3 fatty acids help support heart and brain health). Using plenty of herbs and spices while embracing the Mediterranean diet not only adds flavor and anti-inflammatory properties to foods, but it helps cut down on the need for salt.

The plan limits red meat consumption and replaces butter with healthier fats, such as olive oil. (Olive oil and nuts are wonderful sources of monounsaturated fats; they help lower blood cholesterol levels, and thus the risk of heart disease and stroke.) It gives a nod to drinking red wine (in moderation) and a big plug for physical activity. And, critical to this lifestyle, the Mediterranean diet emphasizes enjoyable meals with family and friends.

Research continues to evaluate the mechanisms by which the Mediterranean diet supports health. What is clear is that it's a synergistic effect, not one particular food, that provides the benefits.

"BAD" CARBS

All that sounds good, but aren't carbohydrates bad for you? How can they be the key to a centenarian diet? People have heard so much negative press about these foods that they don't even ask about cutting them out of their diets—they just do it.

Last year, I received a call from a cardiologist's office. The doctor had referred to me a sixty-seven-year old man with a history of heart disease and a new diagnosis of prediabetes. By the time I met with Larry, he had cut most starches out of his diet. As a result, his diet skewed way too high in protein and fats. Larry enjoyed running and weightlifting, but he needed a lot of convincing to start adding the right carbs to support both his athletic and medical needs.

To be honest, many carbohydrate foods are not healthy for us. For example, we over-consume "white" foods, those with white flour that are high in sugar and fat, and low in dietary fiber. In fact, my oldest daughter was recently diagnosed with gestational diabetes. The first advice she received: Stop eating all foods with white flour. Cakes, cookies, sugary breakfast cereals, and white bread lead this category.

I think we healthcare professionals inadvertently heralded in the problem with the "wrong" carbs a couple of decades ago when we pushed the Food Guide Pyramid as the model for healthy eating. At the bottom of the pyramid, forming the base for a good diet, was the Bread, Cereal, Rice, and Pasta group, from which you were to eat 6-11 servings daily. While we were helping people figure out how to get so many starches in their diets, we didn't do an adequate job of promoting healthy, high-fiber carbohydrates. So people were just eating a lot of "carbs."

Even before this situation, Dr. Atkins' low-carb, high-protein diet was very popular. I'll talk more about low-carb diets and weight loss in another chapter, but this plan was extremely limited in all carbohydrates, and not appropriate for many people.

And then we had the low-fat craze, when food manufacturers were cranking out tasty foods to meet this bill. Remember Nabisco SnackWells in the 1990s? These were "healthy" low-fat cookies that consumers couldn't get enough off. I can recall not being able to find our favorite chocolate variety because they flew off the shelves so quickly. A closer look at the label revealed the first ingredient in these goodies was unbleached enriched flour followed by a couple of forms of sugar.

It turns out that to make a low-fat product tasty, you have to put a lot of sugar in it, with no dietary fiber, creating a cookie that's far from "healthy." Meanwhile, Americans got fatter and chronic diseases soared.

EXERCISE

Which carbohydrate foods do you believe you should be eliminating or limiting in a healthy diet? These could be crackers, cookies, fruits, vegetables, rice, pasta, breads, cereals, or crackers.

_____

_____

_____

_____

_____

GOOD CARBS

So now we nutritionists are fighting an uphill battle to educate people about the role carbohydrates play in a healthy eating plan. We're talking specifically about carbs high in _dietary fiber_, a diet component very misunderstood based on my conversations with family members and clients.

Just what is dietary fiber, why is it important, and how much should you consume? Dietary fiber, also known as "roughage," is the part of a plant that we humans cannot completely digest and absorb. As a result, it passes through the GI tract relatively intact and leaves the body.

Dietary fiber is only found in plant products, most notably whole grains, legumes and dried beans, nuts, fruits, and vegetables. It is not found in meats of any kind.

Two types of dietary fiber exist: soluble and insoluble. _Soluble_ fiber, found in oats, peas, beans, fruit, and barley, dissolves in water. It binds with cholesterol and actually escorts the "bad" variety out of the body, *lowering blood cholesterol levels and the risk of heart attacks*. Soluble fiber also helps *lower the risk of diabetes*; because it isn't absorbed, it doesn't cause spikes in blood sugar levels, decreasing swings in insulin and glucose.

Insoluble fiber promotes the movement of food through your digestive system and adds bulk to your stool, *helping relieve constipation*. This type of fiber is found in whole wheat, wheat bran, nuts, seeds, and some vegetables.

Many plant products contain both soluble and insoluble fiber.

High-fiber foods are generally more filling than low-fiber ones and may aid in losing weight. You can actually fill up on these without feeling hungry quickly. So eating a high-fiber diet can help control weight and reduce the risk of cardiovascular disease; for that reason, the American Heart Association recommends this eating pattern. A high-fiber diet can also help control blood sugar (glucose), which is why the American Diabetes Association recommends it. And these foods can help you live longer; a 2014 analysis of seventeen studies concluded that for every additional ten grams of fiber consumed, the risk of death decreased by 10 percent.[9]

But the most exciting research for Baby Boomers and older adults is that a high-fiber diet may be the key to aging without disabling diseases. A 2016 study published in the *Journal of Gerontology*[10] followed more than 1,600 adults, aged forty-nine and over, for ten years. The researchers were studying successful aging, defined as "absence of disability, depressive symptoms, cognitive impairment, respiratory symptoms, and chronic diseases (eg, cancer and coronary artery disease)."

Of all the variables they followed, researchers found a high-fiber diet led to the highest chance of "reaching old age disease free and fully functional." That is significant information!

EXERCISE

Which high-fiber foods do you currently eat? Think about all meals, including snacks.

1. _____

2. _____

3. _____

4. _____

5. _____

6. _____

7. _____

8. _____

9. _____

10. _____

GETTING TO THIRTY-EIGHT

If a plant-based diet is healthy, just how much dietary fiber is needed to attain the benefits of a healthy plant-based diet? And how does one possibly get to those numbers?

The Institutes of Medicine recommend that men consume thirty-eight grams of dietary fiber per day; the amount for women is twenty-five.[11] Most Americans consume half that amount, about fifteen grams per day.

When I first started working with Peter, he found that listing his food intake in the online program MyFitnessPal helped him track and monitor calories and nutrients. One component we looked at every week was dietary fiber; the program set his goal appropriately at thirty-eight grams per day. Peter looked at his "regular" diet and couldn't imagine eating that much fiber. But with careful planning and education, he was eventually able to select low-calorie, high-fiber foods to fit the bill.

Here are a few guidelines to help you get to your fiber numbers:

- First, read labels. For grain products such as bread, cereal, or crackers, you want the first ingredient to contain the word "whole." So you're looking for "whole wheat" or "whole grain." Next, check on the Nutrition Facts for "Carbohydrates." Then look farther down for "Dietary Fiber." For a food to be considered a good source of dietary fiber, it must contain 2.5 grams per serving.
- Second, dried beans and peas are excellent sources of dietary fiber, many containing ten-plus grams per cup.
- Third, whole fruits and vegetables with skin are also great sources, especially berries, pears, apples, artichokes, and broccoli.

Important note: Ease slowly into a high-fiber diet. Consuming too much of this dietary component too quickly can lead to GI distress such as gas and cramping.

A list of high-fiber foods and a sample menu are at the back of this book in Special Reports.

NUDGING YOURSELF INTO A PLANT-BASED DIET

Can't imagine decreasing your meat intake? Wondering how to

find non-meat entrées? Think you won't feel full after eating? Here are some suggestions to start you on your plant-based journey.

1. Begin by decreasing your portion size of meat, especially at dinnertime. Again, a three-ounce serving—the size of a deck of cards—is all that's needed.

2. Stop building meals around meat; it should only occupy one-quarter of your plate. Half your plate should be filled with fruits and vegetables.

3. Add vegetables into meat entrées, such as grated zucchini and carrots in spaghetti sauce or meatloaf.

4. Look to other cuisines—Mexican, Italian, Greek, and Asian—for non-meat ideas.

5. Experiment with plant sources of protein such as pinto or black beans, lentils, or nuts.

6. Try Meatless Mondays: Designate one day per week when you have vegetarian meals.

EXERCISE

List ten ways you can start concentrating on a plant-based diet.

1. _____

2. _____

3. _____

4. _____

5. _____

6. _____

7. _____

8. _____

9. _____

10. _____

SUMMARY

The evidence is clear that our eating habits influence our possibility of developing chronic disease and, thus, reducing our quality of life and longevity. And a plant-based diet, as seen in the Blue Zones and Mediterranean diet, *will* support physical and mental health as we age.

Research relates these eating patterns to a longer life with the absence of disability and chronic disease, including high blood pressure, heart attack and heart disease, type 2 diabetes, and possibly Alzheimer's.

A diet to support healthy aging includes loading up on high-fiber foods such as whole grains, legumes and dried beans, nuts, seeds, fruits, and vegetables; eating a small amount of meat (a three-ounce portion no more than once a week), fish twice weekly, a small glass of red wine (full of antioxidant polyphenols and the flavonoid resveratrol, which may help increase good cholesterol and decrease bad cholesterol), and moderate amounts of low-fat or fat-free dairy products.

Concentrating on these healthy high-fiber carbs—not processed, sweetened "white" versions—is key. Our bodies do not fully digest and absorb dietary fiber, so depending on the type, that fiber can help usher bad cholesterol out of the body and modulate swings in blood glucose (sugar) and insulin, decreasing the risk of heart disease and diabetes, respectively. A high-fiber diet also helps us stay fuller longer, aiding in weight control.

To get started on your plant-focused diet, look at food labels for good sources of dietary fiber and plan your dinner plate to contain the following: one half fruits and vegetables, one quarter whole grains, one quarter protein. Experiment with ways to add veggies and non-meat protein sources to your entrées, and get inspired by ethnic meals that feature many vegetarian ideas.

Like healthy older adults around the globe, choose veggies, fruits, whole grains, legumes, dried peas and beans, nuts, and seeds for you and your family.

CHAPTER 6

MAXIMIZING FRUIT AND VEGETABLE INTAKE

"We should all be eating fruits and vegetables as if
our lives depend on it—because they do."

— Michael Greger

Eating the right foods is key to living life fully, especially as we age. And that means concentrating primarily on a plant-based diet with whole foods prepared at home. This throws the responsibility for our wellness squarely at our own doorsteps. But it doesn't have to be difficult, and it doesn't have to be expensive. Commitment and planning are the keys.

The cornerstone for a healthy diet is eating an abundance of fruits and vegetables. I like to tell my clients to "eat the rainbow"! That is, consume lots of produce in all colors—red, orange, yellow, green, blue, and purple. Although some items in this category have been tagged "super foods," it's more important to eat a variety of items from these groups. We'll discuss the details in this chapter.

THIS OLD ADVICE IS STILL GOOD

You hear a lot about eating fruits and vegetables, but why are they so important, how much is enough, and how do we possibly get that much into a daily diet? Today, many people ask me these questions, and together, we come up with workable solutions.

I remember when I first started paying attention to nutrition advice—it was in 1977 after college. I was working at a hospital in Dayton, Ohio, completing my dietetic internship. This would be the first time I went to professional meetings and heard speakers in the healthcare field, and the first time I started educating patients about food guidelines.

It was at one of these lectures that I heard a piece of advice that still holds true today—forty years later. (That's impressive in the dynamic field of nutrition, where discoveries and recommendations change often.) The speaker was quoting the American Cancer Society in addressing dietary measures to avoid cancer. At that time, the society's advice was that one of the best ways to protect yourself from cancer was to eat five servings of fruits and vegetables per day.

I remember thinking that sounded too simple; you couldn't possibly keep that terrible disease at bay by eating produce. However, as years passed and researchers uncovered the powerhouse potential of these foods, it became clear fruits and vegetables are indeed critical not only for cancer prevention, but for thwarting other chronic diseases as well.

As I've worked with clients over the years, I've learned that fruits and vegetables are not only misunderstood, but they're under-consumed and sometimes completely ignored. As a result, I often toil to find ways for people to work these foods into their daily eating patterns.

EXERCISE

Think of a typical week. What specific fruits and vegetables do you eat, how often, and how much? Do you have a lot of variety, or (as most people I know) do you consume the same limited ones every day?

_____

_____

_____

_____

_____

_____

_____

_____

_____

THE SECRET LIVES OF FRUITS AND VEGETABLES

Okay, what's all the fuss about an apple or a piece of broccoli? Why not just take a vitamin pill? I hear these questions often, so before I get into how much we should be eating, I think it's important to understand why these foods have become the foundation for a healthy diet to support aging.

Again, going back many years, when I was growing up, we learned that fruits and vegetables were good sources of vitamins. Oranges provided vitamin C that kept scurvy at bay (wasn't important to me) and carrots prevented night blindness (didn't know anybody with that problem). We also learned this category of foods supplies vitamin A, B vitamins (especially folic acid), and vitamin K.

These foods also contain many vital minerals. A few of these include iron, magnesium, potassium, calcium, sodium, and zinc. And fruits and veggies constitute one of the Four Food Groups we learned about back in the '60s—just one part of a healthy diet.

Then dietary fiber started to rise to prominence; fruits and vegetables are excellent sources of this dietary component. In Chapter 5, we learned how fiber plays a role in weight management, as well as in decreasing the risk of heart disease, type 2 diabetes, and other chronic diseases because of the "roughage" these foods contain.

But the most exciting research about fruits and vegetables centers around food components called *phytochemicals*. These are naturally-occurring chemicals that plants produce; they provide the plants with their characteristic colors, odors, and flavors. For example, they're what make blueberries blue and give chili peppers their bite.

Phytochemicals are not essential, so they're not considered to be nutrients like vitamins and minerals. And we don't seem to have long-term storage capacity in our bodies for them. Their absorption is affected by the microbes in your gut and by your genetics.

Researchers have discovered thousands of these compounds and believe there are many more to be identified. You may be familiar with some popular ones: flavonoids (black tea, berries, parsley), carotenoids (carrots and cantaloupe), curcumin (turmeric), and resveratrol (grapes and wine).

In a recent article in *Today's Dietitian*, the author lays out the benefits of phytochemicals.[1] These compounds can reduce inflammation (anti-inflammatory properties), reduce the risk of oxidative damage to cells (antioxidants), stimulate the immune system, prevent toxic substances in the diet from becoming carcinogenic, prevent DNA damage, aid DNA repair, and activate insulin receptors.

As a result, evidence exists that consuming foods rich in phytochemicals may reduce the risk of:

* cardiovascular disease

* breast, lung, and colon cancer

* Type 2 diabetes

* Alzheimer's and Parkinson's disease

But the author of this article concludes, "Research strongly suggests that consuming foods rich in phytochemicals provides health benefits, but not enough information exists to make specific recommendations for phytochemical intake."

However, scientists and healthcare practitioners do recommend we depend on whole foods, not supplements, for phytochemicals. That's because these compounds co-exist in synergistic relationships in specific proportions we can't adequately reproduce, and there are likely other phytochemicals we haven't discovered yet.

So it's best to include all the colors of the rainbow, as I mentioned before, including berries, cherries, citrus fruits, stone fruits (apricots, peaches), prunes, spinach, broccoli, sweet corn, and tomatoes. Even white-colored produce, including apples, cauliflower, and potatoes, are valuable sources of antioxidants and anti-inflammatories.

WHAT'S RECOMMENDED; WHAT WE ACTUALLY EAT

Now that I've convinced you that fruits and vegetables are a critical part of a longevity diet, just how much do you need to consume? How well are you, and we, as a nation, doing in reaching those goals?

About the second week of working with new clients, I ask them to keep a Food Diary—recording everything they eat and drink, along with amounts—for three days. This gives me a basis from which to make suggestions and gauge success.

I remember the first time I looked at Betty's records. Betty was eighty and less than two months post-open heart surgery when I met her. A widow, she had a poor appetite and had lost weight and muscle strength since her surgery. I couldn't find any fruits she consumed, and her "veggies" were limited to those in mixed dishes her daughter made (for example, turkey chili or split pea soup) and an occasional restaurant appetizer. She stated she didn't like any fruit and was "okay" with some vegetables.

Over the course of a few months, we worked to find a few acceptable additions: melon for breakfast, raisins for snacks, and salads at lunch or dinner. Betty made small changes to her diet, and she was able to start working toward her fruit and veggie goals, even living alone at her age.

As it turns out, Betty is just like the majority of Americans when it comes to the intake of fruits and vegetables. Currently, the 2015-2020 Dietary Guidelines for Americans[2] recommends a daily consumption of 2½ cups of veggies per day, and 2 cups of fruits. Echoing these amounts, the American Institute for Cancer Research[3] recommends at least 3½ to 6 cups of fruits and veggies per day.

However, only about one in ten Americans eats enough of these foods, according to the Centers for Disease Control and Prevention.[4]

Clearly, we have room for improvement. Where do you stand on your consumption of these healthful foods?

EXERCISE

Going back to the list you made earlier in this chapter, and considering that a serving of most fruits is either a whole fruit or half a cup of a canned fruit, and for most vegetables is equal to a ½ cup cooked vegetable or 1 cup raw veggies (such as spinach), how many servings per day do you currently consume?

_____

Note: Some people are concerned about the sugar content of fruits and its implication on our health. This sugar, known as fructose, is naturally occurring. And for most people, it is not a problem: We don't eat enough fruit to get too much fructose; fruits are full of fiber, which slows the digestion and absorption of the natural sugars, and as a result, fruits don't cause big spikes in insulin or blood sugar.

(Having said this, I have to acknowledge that my mother-in-law first discovered she had type 2 diabetes after "overdosing" on a small bag of fresh cherries one spring. I did say this sugar is safe "for most people," so please use common sense.)

Fruit juices have concentrated amounts of fructose and don't require the same time to chew and enjoy, so it's too easy to over-consume these products. I recommend my clients avoid fruit juice, enjoying whole fruits instead.

One final note about the amount of fruits and vegetables to consume: A 2017 study found that, while current fruit and vegetable recommendations do provide protection against disease, the greatest health benefits came from eating *ten portions* per day, or about twice the current recommendation.[5] Researchers at Imperial College London analyzed ninety-five studies on fruit and vegetable intake, involving up to 2 million people world-wide. They believe a total of *7.8 million premature deaths could be prevented worldwide, along with reductions in heart disease, stroke, and cancer, if everyone ate ten portions daily.*

Clearly, increasing fruit and vegetable intake will benefit health, especially as you age.

VEGGIES FOR BREAKFAST? LET'S GET CREATIVE

So now the real work begins, as we go back to one of the first questions in this chapter: How do you possibly consume five to ten servings of fruits and vegetables per day? The answer: You get creative.

So let's start at breakfast. Since I'm not recommending juice, how can you get one of your servings out of the way first thing in the morning? Here are some ideas:

- Mix spinach, onions, or grated zucchini into your scrambled eggs.
- Sprinkle strawberries on your Greek or soy yogurt or cottage cheese.
- Add sliced peaches on top of your whole-wheat pancakes or waffles.
- Top your high-fiber, low-sugar hot or cold cereal with blueber-ries.
- Explore frozen fruit; it's usually packed at peak season with nu-trition content comparable to fresh fruit, and it lasts longer. Use any amount whenever needed.

- For my favorite breakfast, I put half a cup of canned pumpkin on my cooked oatmeal, along with pumpkin pie seasoning and one tablespoon of protein powder. The oats and pumpkin add lots of fiber to stabilize blood sugar.

Snacks are a great way to meet your fruit and veggie numbers. Many of my clients can't get all their fruit and veggie servings in their meals, so we add them between meals. Eat them with a small protein source, such as a handful of nuts. Here are some great snack tips:

- Keep small containers of dried fruit on hand so you can grab them when you rush out the door. (Note: Dried fruit is high in sugar and calories, so keep it to a minimum if you're trying to lose weight.)
- Keep a bowl of fruit in prominent view in your kitchen. Fill it with bananas, apples, and oranges. You're much more likely to grab fruit if you don't have to go looking for it.
- Buy baby carrots and keep your favorite hummus or low-calorie ranch dressing on hand.

Use lunch as a way to get creative when adding vegetables. Here's how:

- Add avocado, spinach, tomatoes, or green pepper slices to your sandwich. Think about the array of veggies you see at your local sandwich shop, and create your own tasty, healthy sub.
- Add diced apple and celery to your tuna salad.
- Top salads with dried cranberries, strawberries, or orange slices.
- Enjoy a homemade smoothie with handfuls of spinach, a very ripe banana for sweetening, and any other produce you like, along with water or milk, and yogurt or a scoop of protein powder.

- Along with carrots, use sliced celery, zucchini, or cucumber with peanut butter or your favorite healthy dip.

- If you're preparing food for somebody else (spouse or grand-child), do some extra work before serving. While it takes a couple of minutes to peel an orange or slice an apple, most people are more likely to consume produce if it's served "ready to eat."

Finish your day with your plate half-full of veggies and fruit for dinner. Here's how:

- Follow the same guidelines as above for lunch.

- Grate carrots and zucchini into mixed dishes like casseroles or spaghetti sauce; sauté first with onions.

- Add canned pumpkin to red sauce dishes like chili and spaghetti sauce. Pumpkin thickens the product, cuts acidic taste, and adds lots of fiber and phytochemicals.

- Make a meal with homemade soups—butternut squash and split pea are favorites of mine.

- Visit the pre-cut section of your produce aisle. These pre-cut mixtures of fresh vegetables, often mixed in with herbs, are good for a couple of servings. While at first glance it seems these items cost too much, my clients remind me that if you're cooking for just one or two, and you buy a full bag of spinach or a whole zucchini, there's a good chance you'll end up throwing away some of it. Also, they're worth a look if you have problems slicing or chopping your own foods. So explore the pre-cut items and make your own determination.

- Purchase a salad from your grocery store salad bar area and bring it home. You can use the items in your to-go container to cook or snack on later.

- Make your own ethnic "bowl" with a base of brown rice. Add canned black or pinto beans (low-sodium varieties are available), diced tomatoes and onions, corn, and chopped romaine or spinach. Be creative with these.

- Investigate plain frozen vegetables; they're a nutrition bargain like frozen fruit. Avoid "seasoned" veggies or those in sauces to keep the sodium and calorie intake down.

- Canned vegetables are another possibility; again, watch the sodium amount. Check the Nutrition Facts label and pick the item with the least sodium. You can also rinse canned vegetables to reduce salt content.

- Have a ripe, in-season piece of fruit for dessert with a small square of dark chocolate.

EXERCISE

Go through each meal, and at least one snack, and write out the fruits and vegetables you will eat. List at least three different possibilities per meal.

_____

_____

_____

_____

_____

_____

_____

SUMMARY

Eating an abundance of fruits and vegetables is key to enhancing your body's natural ability to fight disease. While most Americans do not eat the recommended number of servings (a minimum of about five per day), strong evidence exists that fruits and vegetables' fiber and phytochemical content will help us live out a long, healthy life.

It's important to consume a variety of fruits and vegetables. They all contain different vitamins, minerals, dietary fibers, and phytochemicals in specific amounts and combinations that support wellness. So don't depend on supplements—eat your produce in all colors.

While 5-10 servings per day can be a challenge, get creative and think outside the dinner plate to fulfill your daily fruit and veggie goals. Leafy greens go well with eggs for breakfast, sandwiches can be topped with crunchy vegetables, and the frozen section of your grocery store might be an excellent place to explore produce that will last longer than a week. Snack time is great for munching on carrot sticks and peanut butter, or grabbing an extra apple or bunch of grapes. And finally, fill half of your plate at dinner with vegetables and fruit, cooked or raw. If you eat canned fruit, be sure it's packed without added sugar; select canned veggies with the lowest sodium content.

Eat the "rainbow" of fruits and vegetables every day and look forward to a long life, knowing you're helping your body guard against chronic diseases.

CHAPTER 7

CONCENTRATING ON WHOLE FOODS, PREPARED AT HOME

"Don't eat anything your great-grandmother wouldn't recognize as food."

— Michael Pollan

We've now talked about the importance of a plant-based diet, highlighting ways to get more fruits and vegetables into your diet. These foods are critical for supporting a healthy heart, immune system, and brain, especially as we age.

It's equally important, as reflected in lessons from the Blue Zones, to depend on meals prepared at home. Unfortunately, processed foods now make up approximately 70 percent of the American diet.[1] It's been a gradual shift over the past 100 years, but one that we can personally change to improve our health.

PROCESSED FOODS AND YOUR METABOLISM

Is your diet full of these foods? Do you just open a container and heat your meal in the microwave, as opposed to chopping and cooking your own foods? Do you go from high-sugar, low-fiber cereal to white bread with processed cheese and luncheon meats to frozen dinners and cookies throughout the day?

Would you be so eager to eat this way if you knew this trend was making you fatter and less healthy?

Processed items are foods that have been cooked, canned, frozen, or packaged, and often even changed in nutritional composition by fortifying or preserving. However, let me say right now that not all processed foods are "bad." For example, bagged green salads are "processed," as is yogurt. But other items are less healthy. Ready-to-eat foods—ones that require no cooking before consuming such as crackers, cereal, and luncheon meats—can be less wholesome. Pre-made meals, such as frozen and microwaveable dinners, are highly processed and not the best choices for our wellbeing.

We often interchange the word "processed" with "convenience" or "junk" food when thinking about items that are no longer as nutritionally sound as the original food. Think of French fries versus a potato or white bread versus whole-grain bread. These foods are often high in calories and additives.

Because processed foods account for such a high proportion of our dietary intake, and because obesity has also risen in the past fifty-plus years, researchers have speculated there may be a connection between these two trends. To test this theory, a small study evaluated the relationship between processed foods and our metabolism, or the rate at which we burn calories after a meal.[2]

Researchers found the energy expenditure after eating processed food was almost *50 percent less* than from less-processed foods. Seems it may just take more energy to digest and metabolize whole foods compared to processed ones.

Can you imagine how much more weight you might accumulate if you eat mainly processed foods?

EXERCISE

Take an inventory of the foods you eat on a daily basis. Write down everything from each meal, including entrées, drinks, desserts, and snacks. How many of these are processed foods?

_____

_____

_____

_____

_____

_____

_____

_____

_____

_____

SUGARS AND SODIUM AND FATS, OH MY!

Processed foods generally taste so good that we Americans are addicted to them. But just what are we trading for flavor and convenience?

Many processed foods are high in added sugar. Sugar is used to make foods taste better, to increase the browning and improve the texture of baked items, and to preserve foods. It's found in everything from breads to catsup and soda. The more foods you prepare from scratch, the more you control the amount of sugar in your diet—and your body will thank you.

Processed foods are also high in sodium, one of two components that make up salt. Like sugar, sodium enhances flavor, preserves freshness, and improves the texture and appearance of foods. According to the Centers for Disease Control and Prevention, 75 percent of the sodium in our diet comes from restaurant, pre-packaged, and processed foods, *not salt you add to foods*.[3] A frozen microwaveable meal can contain up to 1,800 mg of sodium; a whopping amount compared to the recommendation of no more than 2,300 mg per day. While we do need a certain amount of sodium in our diets, too much can be a problem.

Fats are added to food to help make them shelf-stable and improve texture; unfortunately, they also increase calories. In some cases, these are trans fats or saturated fats, which, if consumed in large amounts, can have a negative effect on blood lipids (fats), increasing the risk of heart attack and stroke.

Artificial additives are chemicals whose names you can't pronounce and don't recognize, but which are also prevalent in processed foods. They add a specific color, preserve foods, and/or enhance a flavor or texture. Some studies show these chemicals can be harmful; others do not. Clearly, the more homemade foods you eat, the less of these chemicals you will consume.

One final note about what's *missing* in many highly refined foods: dietary fiber. In the processing of wheat, the healthful bran and wheat germ are often processed out. We've already talked about the importance of dietary fiber, and the fact that a "good source" is a level of at least 2.5 grams per serving. A glance at the Nutrition Facts label on foods like many ready-to-eat cereals, breakfast bars, muffins, cookies, and others reveals low dietary fiber amounts.

SOME "PROCESSING" IS GOOD

In reality, any time we cook, peel, or even chop foods, we're "processing" them. Is there, then, a place in a wholesome diet for some of these items?

Most experts do, in fact, agree that some processing is acceptable. For example, canned items such as vegetables (you can rinse these to lower sodium content) or fruit packed in juice or water are healthy choices. And processing actually improves the nutritional impact of others foods. Dairy products have added calcium and vitamin D (to enhance the absorption of calcium), and in the milling of grains, cooking generally increases digestibility of nutrients.

So there is definitely a place for some processed foods in a healthy diet:

- plain frozen fruits and vegetables
- pre-cut veggies
- canned fruits (no sugar added)
- canned vegetables and legumes, including pinto, black, and garbanzo beans (check for lowest sodium choice)

- whole-grain bread products

- brown rice and quinoa

- whole-grain pasta

- low-sugar, high-fiber fortified breakfast cereals

- plain oatmeal

- veggie burgers (watch the sodium amount)

- dried fruits (can be high in sugar and calories, but also high in key nutrients and fiber; eat in moderation)

- peanut or almond butter (with no added sugar or fats; look for "natural" on the label)

- string cheese or plain yogurt (vegan varieties are available)

- fermented foods such as sauerkraut, kimchi, or kefir

- teas

- coffee—"black" is best

- dark chocolate, at least 70 percent cacao—my go-to dessert (one small square, 62.5 calories); this indulgence contains the phytochemical flavonoid, found to lower cholesterol and blood pressure levels

But eat with caution highly processed foods such as potato chips, low-fiber, white flour grain products (muffins, cookies, cakes, many ready-to-eat breakfast cereals), frozen and microwavable meals, cured meats, soft drinks, fast foods, and restaurant meals.

WHOLE FOODS, PREPARED AT HOME

I have lots of fond food memories from my childhood. We loved watching our mother create homemade jam from our backyard apricots. I remember my father coming home after work and tend-ing our large vegetable garden, bringing in his bounty of home-grown artichokes, green beans, and other produce. Our Aunt Virginia spent hours in the kitchen, surrounded by family and love, creating traditional Italian dishes we couldn't wait to eat.

How can we realistically get back to those whole foods, prepared at home? It's not as difficult as you may think. Let's explore some ideas.

For the purpose of this discussion, I'll define "whole" foods as those as close to their natural state as possible, still in their recognizable forms, and full of nutrients like dietary fiber and phytochemicals. And because many of my clients are concerned about money and the amount of time it takes to stand and prepare homemade recipes, I'll keep these parameters in mind, also.

So here are some of my best suggestions to incorporate whole foods into your diet:

1. Plan your meals in advance, and shop with a list. Start with fresh fruits and vegetables, along with the foods "bulleted" in the list above.

2. Plant a vegetable or herb garden, find or start a community garden, or shop from your local farmer's market.

3. Purchase dry items in bulk (pasta, rice, spices).

4. Ease into whole foods by combining them with convenience items. For example, add your own diced or grated veggies to seasoning mixes of spaghetti, chili, or stew.

5. Designate one evening or weekend day to prepare meals you can eat throughout the week.

6. Team up with a family member or friend who loves to cook. Offer to buy the food and provide wine or dessert in exchange for him or her coming over and preparing dinner occasionally.

7. Cook multiple portions of foods and store for later. For example, bake several chicken breasts and use for meals over several days. Hard-boil multiple eggs and store refrigerated for up to one week. Make a big pot of soup and enjoy over several days.

8. Make large portions of cold items. You can prepare a gigantic salad, store it without salad dressing, and enjoy it over several days. Try making two sandwiches at one time, and refrigerate one for later. (Don't add wet ingredients like tomatoes until you're ready to eat the second sandwich.)

9. Buy nuts in bulk and place in small plastic bags for quick snacks.

10. Eat fresh fruit in season for dessert.

11. Use baked potatoes or sweet potatoes as a base for a meal. Different healthy toppings for them include steamed veggies, homemade chili, spaghetti sauce, or nuts.

12. Add fresh or frozen fruit to plain Greek or vegan yogurt.

13. Purchase "minimally processed" foods with five ingredients or less.

14. Follow the advice from food behavior researcher Brian Wansink of Cornell University. He's discovered simple ways we can encourage better eating, an approach he's coined as the "C.A.N." method.[4] Make healthy foods "convenient" so they're easy to see and consume. Make these items "attractive" in appearance. And finally, make consuming them "normal." Some examples of this method include: Place healthy foods within easy reach while "hiding" unhealthy items at the back of shelves or in difficult-to-reach places. Display fruit in an attractive bowl, as mentioned in the previous chapter.

Instead of buying grapes and hiding them in a refrigerator drawer, rinse them when you get home from the store, cut big bunches into smaller ones, and place them on the middle shelf of the refrigerator (not hidden in a drawer) where you'll be reminded to grab them more often! Model good eating habits for others, especially children.

EXERCISE

List ten whole foods you will buy, along with ways to encourage their consumption.

_____

_____

_____

_____

_____

_____

_____

_____

_____

_____

SUMMARY

Processed foods far outweigh whole foods in terms of what Americans eat, but they are simply not the healthiest choices. These items are often full of sugar, sodium, and unhealthy fats, and they lack naturally-occurring nutrients such as dietary fiber and phytochemicals.

Granted, eating healthful, whole foods can be a challenge. Price, preparation, and even taste may discourage people from purchasing these items. But with a little planning, we can not only stock up on these foods, but employ methods to encourage us to eat more of them. (Yes, you C.A.N.).

And the payoff from eating better can add years to your life.

A 2017 study published in the *New England Journal of Medicine* followed nearly 74,000 Americans for twelve years.[5] Researchers found that improved diet quality over the study period was consistently associated with a *decreased risk of death*. People who added more fruits, vegetables, whole grains, fish, low-fat dairy, and "good" fats such as olive oil and nuts outlived those who ate more processed foods, sweets, red meat, and butter.

Another important note from this study: Most of the participants were sixty years old or older.

So no excuses. Take stock of what you're eating—look in your cupboards, refrigerator, and freezer, and scrutinize your grocery shopping receipts. Then find ways to create healthy substitutions and make them easy to consume.

It's never too late to adopt better eating habits, and you may be rewarded with a longer, healthier life.

CHAPTER 8

PUSHING AND PULLING—CHALLENGING FOR STRENGTH

"Eating alone will not keep a man well.
He must also take exercise."

— Hippocrates

Up to this point, we've mainly discussed the importance of diet in our journey toward aging with strength and independence. The emphasis must be on plant-based foods with plenty of fruits and vegetables, in forms we still recognize. Meals prepared at home with whole foods provide the best chance to control what goes into our bodies, and what we keep out.

I've also emphasized why we need to keep moving throughout the day, every day. Too much sedentary time is associated with a host of chronic diseases.

In this chapter, we'll examine why strength training is vital for maintaining the quality of life we desire in our seventies, eighties, nineties, and beyond. Picking up weights is not a likely consideration for most folks as they age, but one we must begin to embrace. It's a major factor in the growing realization that exercise is a potent preventive medicine, safer and more effective than any drug you can take.

WHY PUMP IRON?

I recently was interviewed on a late night health radio show. One of the questions the host asked was: Which is more important as we age, our diet or exercise? That took a moment of thought before I answered because the truth is they're both critical. Without fuel, our bodies won't function properly. But without strong muscles to allow us to walk, feed ourselves, or to pick us up off the ground after a fall, food loses its importance.

Have you ignored exercise as you've gotten older, especially strength training?

I've met many people who believe that walking and working out occasionally with light weights is all the exercise they need. These folks are often surprised to find out how much muscle they've lost and how much fat they've gained as they've gotten older. It was especially surprising to my clients Larry and Catherine, a husband and wife who exercised regularly. Unfortunately, unhealthy percentages of body fat and an evaluation of their strength training regimen suggested they were not working out as effectively as they could.

Let's make sure you don't misinterpret the above paragraph. *Walking is vital for keeping us healthy*, as I'll explain in the following chapter. But you must *also strengthen and build muscles if you want a truly independent and self-sustaining life.*

From our thirties on, we begin to lose 3-5 percent of our muscle mass per decade. That means sedentary adults can lose 15-25 percent of the total number of fibers in their muscles by the time they are eighty. This process is called *sarcopenia*, and it leads to loss of strength, balance, mobility, and independence.

Strength training, along with proper diet, is the only known intervention to protect against age-related muscle loss.

And as we lose muscle, our metabolism goes down. As a result, our bodies need fewer calories and we're more likely to gain weight, especially excess body fat, unless caloric intake is reduced. So even if you happen to weigh the same at seventy as you did at twenty-five, if you haven't lifted weights, you have a much higher proportion of body fat compared to muscle. Unfortunately, excess fat can lead to a multitude of health problems.

Think your muscles are still strong enough? Answer these questions related to everyday activities:

- Can you walk up and down a set of stairs?
- Can you get off a chair, sofa, or toilet without pushing with your hands?
- Sit on the floor, in the middle of a room. Pretend you've just fallen. Can you get up without the aid of a chair, sofa, bed, coffee table, or wall? This is something you may need to do at some point.
- Can you carry a bag of groceries?
- Do you lose your balance easily?
- Can you still manage your own luggage?
- Can you open heavy doors?
- Are you still able to play with your grandchildren?

EXERCISE

Take stock of your own strength, honestly. Which activities have become more difficult for you to accomplish? Which ones are critical for maintaining your desired lifestyle?

_____

_____

_____

_____

_____

_____

_____

In addition to maintaining independence and strength, weight training helps:[1]

- Strengthen your bones
- Reduce your risk of falling
- Improve control of blood sugar
- Increase your metabolism
- Improve your body composition to less fat and more muscle
- Reduce your resting blood pressure
- Speed up the rate at which food moves through your digestive system, reducing the risk of colon cancer
- Reduce your risk of low back injury
- Elevate your mood and your self-confidence

- Relieve pain from osteoarthritis and rheumatoid arthritis

- Enhance recovery from stroke or heart attack

- Decrease incidence of diabetes and cardiovascular disease. A 2016 study looked at exercise levels of more than 35,000 women aged 47-98, and concluded muscle-strengthening exercises in physical activity regimens were necessary for reduced risk of type 2 diabetes and cardiovascular disease, independent of aerobic exercise.[2]

It may come as a surprise, but strength training is also valuable for your brain and emotional state. Here are a few of the documented benefits:[3]

- Improved memory
- Improved executive control
- May lessen depression
- Much less chronic fatigue
- Improved quality of sleep
- Improved cognition
- Less anxiety
- Improved self-esteem

AREN'T I TOO OLD TO LIFT WEIGHTS?

As a kid in the '60s, I distinctly remember watching Jack LaLanne on our old TV. I was impressed at that time by his various athletic feats, but I was more surprised as the years passed to see the "Godfather of Fitness" continue to weightlift well into older age. He was a pioneer and inspiration, yet many myths about strength training continue to dissuade Baby Boomers and seniors from picking up a set of weights. Given the consequences of sarcopenia and all the benefits of strength training, can you afford *not* to do it?

Let's discuss some of the common misconceptions and questions about building muscles as we age.

1. **I'm too old to gain muscle.** With proper training, it's possible to gain muscle size and strength well into the eighth decade of life.[4] Granted, it's not a fast process. Working out twice a week, it will take 10-12 weeks to see results; that's more time than it takes a younger person, but it's still attainable. I've watched many clients in their seventies and eighties improve both upper and lower body strength while training with me. With Betty, we documented a 233 percent increase in leg strength and 30 percent increase in arm strength over four months using standard assessment tests for older adults. When beginning to lift weights, be patient and consistent, progressively increasing the amount of resistance.

2. **I'm a woman and I don't want to get bulky muscles.** Not to worry. Females don't have enough muscle mass or tissue-building hormones for large, bulky muscles. But you can have strong muscles to help keep you safe and independent.

3. **I have muscle pain after lifting weights; isn't that harmful?** It's perfectly normal to feel muscle pain a day or two after you exercise. It's called DOMS (delayed-onset muscle soreness), and it's caused by exercise-induced microscopic tears in muscle fibers. DOMS usually occurs when an individual begins strength training or increases the intensity/duration of the program. The pain will lessen in a few days. I always warn newcomers to my exercise classes about DOMS, and I encourage them to keep coming back despite the pain. It really does go away with time. Note: If you start to feel *joint* pain, something is wrong; change your exercise routine and see your doctor.

4. **I need special protein drinks to get more muscles.** You do need to eat *enough* protein to build and maintain muscle

mass. While most Americans eat more than enough protein, some seniors don't meet their needs. We'll talk more about protein in Chapter 15, but suffice to say, it's important to get enough high-quality protein throughout the day.

5. **I walk. That's all the exercise I need.** Walking is an extremely valuable activity for folks as we age. But keep this in mind: Both muscle and bone mass decrease with age, and walking does not build muscle size for strong legs nor does it significantly strengthen bones. You must challenge muscles with resistance.

EXERCISE

What are some beliefs you have about strength training that may be keeping you from lifting weights, or performing squats, lunges, or push-ups?

_____

_____

_____

_____

_____

_____

_____

WEIGHT TRAINING: IF I CAN DO IT...

Only about 20 percent of American adults meet the government's recommendation for both cardiovascular and strength training.[5]

I'll talk more about the cardio, or aerobic, guidelines in the next chapter.

The strength-building guidelines are: *Adults perform muscle-strengthening activities of moderate or high intensity and involve all major muscle groups two or more days a week.* These recommendations hold even for older adults.

But how do most adults, who have never lifted a pair of weights and don't own a gym membership, begin to benefit from strength training?

Here's my story. Twelve years ago, when I was fifty-two, my younger daughter graduated from high school, so I was ready for some "me" time! I walked into a gym for the first time. I hired a trainer, eager to get in shape and conquer the skill of strength training. A typical female Baby Boomer, I enjoyed the cardio and weight machines, but I was completely intimidated by the area of the gym I called the "Testosterone Corner." It was where the muscular guys hung out, grunting and grimacing with their dumbbells, barbells, and cable machines. Over the years, with lots of work pushing and pulling weights, this fear has completely disappeared! Not only do I enjoy working out in this area, but I'm completely sold on the critical importance of these exercises.

Here are three lessons I've gleaned from the Testosterone Corner:

1. **Get over yourself!** Really, nobody's staring at you. They're all too busy doing their own thing. Nobody cares which weight you pick up, how many reps you perform, or how your hair looks. And if you have questions, don't be shy—guys (and gals) in this area are happy to help newcomers "learn the ropes."

2. **Use the mirrors!** But don't use them to check out your makeup or clothing. Guys look at themselves all the time in the gym— most likely admiring their bulging muscles. You can definitely

do the same, but mainly use the mirrors to be sure your back is straight, your arms or legs are in the correct place, and your weights are where they're supposed to be.

3. **Don't compare yourselves to others!** You never know how many years somebody's been working out or how many hours he or she spends in the gym, so don't feel bad if others look fitter than you. Concentrate on doing your training, gradually increasing the amount of resistance you can push/pull. And look at the bright side—eventually there will be another person in that area who is even more of a neophyte than you!

BEST PRACTICES

Now it's your turn. Ready to thumb your nose at Mother Nature? Don't forget that in middle age and beyond, it's imperative to start weightlifting *safely*. This is especially critical if you:

- have been sedentary for many years

- are a current or recent smoker

- have a chronic disease (high blood pressure, diabetes, heart disease, arthritis, osteoporosis)

- are overweight/obese

So start your exercise program with safety in mind:

- **Get the approval of your healthcare provider.** Heart conditions, joint problems, bone weakness, blood sugar troubles, and recent surgeries are just a few of the issues that need consideration when starting a fitness program. Make sure your physician evaluates your exercise needs.

- **Review all your meds.** Medications for heart disease, high blood pressure, and diabetes can change your body's response to exercise. Check with your doctor or fitness professional for program modifications and precautions.

Here are some easy ways to get started with strength training. You don't need weights for all exercises, and you don't need a gym membership or specialized equipment.

- Pick up a set of light weights (2 or 3 lbs.) or cans (15 oz.) and simply carry them throughout the house several times per day.

- Perform push-ups against a wall or sturdy countertop. If using a wall, place hands at shoulder height and feet hip-width apart and about 12" from wall. When dropping into the wall, visualize a board that rests on the back of your head, in between your shoulder blades and sits on your tailbone. Don't let your head or chin jut forward; drop into the wall straight like a board.

- Stand up from a chair or sofa without pushing with your arms. That is, just use your leg muscles to get up.

- Sit at the edge of a chair with feet about 12" apart and close to the legs of the chair. Place arms out in front of you. Using your leg muscles, lift your bottom off the chair one or two inches only; then sit back down. Repeat ten times.

Be sure you have plenty of water before, during, and after weight training. And don't exercise on an empty stomach. It's important to eat a protein/carbohydrate food 30-60 minutes after strength training to give your body the building blocks for muscle growth. Half a peanut butter sandwich, string cheese with fruit, or a scoop of protein powder mixed with water will work.

Ready to build muscles? Follow these steps:

1. *Stretching at the right time* is critical. Traditionally, most people stretch before they exercise. While "warming up" is critical before physical activity, especially for folks over fifty, the

type of stretching most people do (holding a "static" stretch in one position without movement) is best performed at the *conclusion of a workout*, when the muscles are properly warmed and, therefore, more pliable.

Prior to strength training, walk for 5-10 minutes to warm up your muscles and get your blood moving.

2. The general guideline is to train all major muscle groups at least twice a week. That means your legs, arms, chest, back, and core. Free weights (dumbbells) work, as do machines at a gym. Machines provide stability and less stress on joints, when used correctly. Take advantage of a free session with a personal trainer when you join an establishment, or read directions posted on the equipment. Incorrect use of any kind of exercise equipment can lead to injury.

    Wait at least forty-eight hours before exercising the same muscles again.

3. Don't hold your breath. Ideally, you exhale as you lift, push, or pull with the weight; inhale as you release the resistance. But just breathe if you get confused.

4. To build strength, you must challenge your muscles. So start with a low weight, one that feels a little difficult but not impossible. When you can perform 10-12 repetitions of an exercise with proper form, add more weight. If using dumbbells, progress from 2 to 3 pounds, or 3 to 4 pounds; if doing exercises on a machine, increase the weight by 10 percent (or as close as possible).

    If you can do at least eight reps at the higher weight, continue working at this level. When you can easily complete twelve reps, move up in weight again.

    Ideally, you want to increase weight about every four weeks.

5. An alternative to lifting heavier weights is to use lighter weights, lifting *until your muscles are exhausted* and you can't do one more repetition.

   Just don't do the same exercises with the same weight in the same order session after session. Mix it up. Challenge your muscles, concentrate on proper form, and get strong!

6. Other methods of strength training include moving your own body weight (push-ups, pull-ups, squats, lunges, sitting and standing many times, jumping), resistance bands and tubing, yoga, tai chi, and Pilates.

EXERCISE

How are you going to strengthen your body? List one method you intend to begin and the date you'll start (after clearing with your doctor). This may be starting a yoga class, buying an exercise CD, using dumbbells and resistance bands and working out at home, joining a gym, or seeking out a class in your community.

_____

_____

_____

_____

_____

_____

_____

SUMMARY

While proper eating will protect you from chronic disease, it will not allow you to *function* in your later years to maintain your quality of life. To live longer and healthier, you must embrace both cardio and strength training because they have different benefits. Strength training, as we discussed in this chapter, is critical for building muscles and strengthening bones, protecting us from injury. It gives us the ability to enjoy cruises, play with grandchildren, and perform all the activities of daily life that allow us to live independently.

Be sure to check with your doctor before beginning a strength-training program. Start with light weights and gradually increase the amount of resistance. If you loathe weightlifting, try using exercise bands/tubing or seek out a yoga, tai chi, or Pilates class. Check with your local YMCA, senior center, parks and recreation department, or even community college for programs you can join.

Find ways to make strength training a habit: do push-ups and squats before breakfast, jump with your grandchildren, lift yourself out of a chair without using your arms, exercise with a buddy, or calendar your workout days at the gym. Your muscles and bones will gain and maintain strength, your body will be protected from chronic diseases, your mood will be elevated, and you'll be better equipped to live the life you desire.

CHAPTER 9

KEEPING YOURSELF HEALTHY WITH CARDIO

"If exercise could be packed in a pill, it would be the single most widely prescribed and beneficial medicine in the nation."

— Robert N. Butler, MD, former director,
National Institute of Aging

If you're looking for independence and quality of life as the years go on, you'll need strong muscles. Strong muscles are supported by strength training—lifting weights, pushing/pulling body weight, or performing activities such as yoga.

But there are two types of exercise critical for healthy aging— strength training *and* cardiovascular (aerobic) exercise. Each type of physical activity supports and complements the other; they offer different benefits.

Before you get upset about fitting even more exercise into your life, here's the good news about cardio: Many activities you already do are categorized as aerobic exercise, and they can be "chunked" down to fit into a busy life. Their life-extending benefits are truly amazing. I'll show you how to take advantage of all they have to offer!

OH, THE '80s! RICHARD SIMMONS AND JANE FONDA MOVED US

Some of my earliest memories of "aerobic" exercise were books, TV shows, and videos back in the '70s and '80s. Jim Fixx had us running. Richard Simmons and Jane Fonda had us rocking and busting our buns to music. We were burning calories and loving it back then. Exercise studios and Jazzercise classes skyrocketed in popularity, and we were out in force with our new water bottles and cute outfits. (I can only speak for us ladies.)

Everybody knew movement was important and healthy for us. But we soon learned we wouldn't benefit from physical activity until we figured out how to make it fun, easy to accomplish, and sustainable—just 51.7 percent of US adults meet the guidelines for aerobic activities.[1]

First, how much do we need and what counts as cardio? If you remember from the previous chapter, the recommendation for muscle strengthening is twice weekly.

> For cardio (officially designated "moderate-to-vigorous physical activity"), the World Health Organization and Centers for Disease Control and Prevention[2] advise: 150 minutes per week, preferably spread throughout the week, or seventy-five minutes of vigorous activity.

Let's break that down. The easiest way to look at that recommendation is thirty minutes of activity, five days per week. If that still sounds intimidating, you can break that thirty minutes down to three ten-minute intervals (perfect if you're still working; use your designated break time for physical activity).

And it doesn't have to be brisk walking, which is an excellent choice for cardio. These activities also count, as long as you can do them at an intensity that increases your heart rate for at least ten minutes.

- walking your dog
- dancing
- swimming/water aerobics
- hiking
- bicycling
- gardening
- playing with your kids/grandchildren
- tennis
- carrying/moving moderate loads (think: groceries)
- housework

EXERCISE

Including walking, what physical activities do you do regularly? Be sure to list "chores" such as vacuuming, washing floors, mowing (no sit-down mowers), picking weeds, and walking your dog. And also think in terms of organized sports. In our area, a sport called pickleball is gaining popularity.

_____

_____

_____

_____

_____

CONQUERING THE "INACTIVITY EPIDEMIC"

We're all growing older; there's just no way to stop the clock. But you don't have to end up like Frank—post-heart attack, obese with high blood pressure, and easily winded with any physical activity, or Sam—unable to lift himself out of a chair and barely able to move about with a walker. Along with poor eating habits, both of these men had suffered from what's been dubbed the "inactivity epidemic," a major public health crisis.

Imagine the power of this new vision, if implemented nationwide: Every time you visit your healthcare provider, you're asked how much you exercise. And then because exercise is designed right into your treatment plan, you leave with a prescription for the appropriate type and amount of physical activity.

This is the national initiative spearheaded by the American College of Sports Medicine (ACSM) called Exercise is Medicine.[3] Recognizing the critical role of regular physical activity in the health of our nation, the underlying principle is to encourage primary care physicians and other healthcare providers to include exercise when designing treatment plans for patients. And it is starting to catch on. My family belongs to Kaiser Permanente in Southern California; we are asked every visit how much we exercise, and I have seen prescription pads for physical activity in exam rooms.

Like strength training, aerobic exercise boasts a long list of benefits,[4] including:

- helps maintain weight loss
- lowers the risk of heart disease and stroke
- lowers the risk of diabetes and metabolic syndrome (combination of too much fat around the waist, high blood pressure, low HDL cholesterol, high triglycerides, or high blood sugar)

- helps lower blood glucose levels in those with diabetes
- lowers the risk of some cancers, including breast and colon cancer
- lowers the risk of having a hip fracture
- helps manage pain and quality of life in those with arthritis
- reduces the risk of developing Alzheimer's disease
- decreases the risk of depression
- helps you sleep better

Still not convinced you need to get up and take that walk or swim? Check out these eye-opening statistics:[5]

- Physical inactivity costs the US healthcare system $330 per person each year, or more than $102 billion dollars annually.
- A low level of physical activity increases the risk of dying *more than* does smoking, obesity, hypertension (high blood pressure), or high cholesterol.
- Active individuals in their eighties have a lower risk of death than inactive individuals in their sixties.
- Regular exercise can be twice as effective in treating type 2 diabetes as the standard insulin prescription and can save $2,250 per person per year when compared to the cost of standard drug treatment.
- Engaging in regular physical activity can decrease depression as effectively as Prozac or behavioral therapy.

Can you afford not to become more physically active?

EXERCISE

Make a list of the chronic health problems you have, or are con-

cerned about "inheriting," that could be avoided or better controlled by exercise. Now write down the "cost" of each condition
(out-of-pocket healthcare dollars, gas or car-related expenses for
medical appointments, medications, or special foods).

_____

_____

_____

_____

_____

_____

_____

CARDIO = BRAIN HEALTH + LONGEVITY

We've known for some time that physical activity helps extend a
healthy life. (In the Blue Zones, centenarians engage regularly in
gardening, walking, hiking, and daily chores.)

Now, research is starting to tell us why. For example, exercise fun-
damentally changes structures in our body that can lead to living
longer with a sharper mind. We'll delve more into this in Chapter 14, but suffice to say that exercise, especially cardio, boosts
the supply of blood and oxygen to the brain and promotes the
growth of natural proteins that help protect it—one of the most
powerful being brain-derived neurotrophic factor (BDNF).

BDNF has been labeled "Miracle Grow for your brain"[6] because
it generates new blood vessels, stimulates new connections between brain cells (neurons), and promotes growth of new neu-

rons (a process called neuroplasticity), especially in areas of the brain related to memory and learning.

Exercise also supports healthy aging by protecting our chromosomes, which shorten and deteriorate with increasing years. In a study published in 2017,[7] exercise accounted for nine years of reduced cellular aging. Another study[8] showed that exercise, especially high-intensity internal training (see below), caused cells to better support the mitochondria (powerhouses where energy is created), and also stopping aging at the cellular level. Both of these studies included groups of older adults.

Now, can you find a few minutes each day—150 per week, which amounts to slightly more than 2 percent of your waking hours—to transform your life into one with greater longevity and vitality?

START WITH SAFETY IN MIND

When I first started working with Betty, I'll admit I was a bit nervous. The scar from her open-heart surgery was still fresh, and she was barely moving with her walker. But she had clearance from her doctor to start exercising, within specified limits, and she was eager to get stronger. Is it safe for you to begin a program of physical activity?

It's worth repeating from the previous chapter, check with your doctor before exercising, especially if you:

• have been sedentary for many years

• are a current or recent smoker

• have a chronic disease (high blood pressure, diabetes, heart disease, arthritis, osteoporosis)

• are overweight/obese

Remember: Although the risks of exercise are small, they do exist for some people, especially those of advancing age. So start off your exercise program gradually. Find a physical activity you enjoy and can visualize continuing for many years. Again, walking, swimming, biking on a flat surface, and yoga are low-impact and help build muscle and stamina without putting excess stress on your body.

Start by doing your physical activity for a few minutes two or three times a week. Increase the number of days you're exercising *before* you increase the amount of time in each session.

If you'll be outside:

- **Check the weather report.** Because an older body doesn't adjust as well to extreme temperatures as it did when it was younger, make sure not to exercise outside in hot or humid weather. On cold days, dress in layers and be sure to cover your fingers, ears, and nose. And if the air quality is poor and you have asthma or other respiratory conditions, avoid physical activity. Drink plenty of water before, during, and after exercise. (Hint: Urine the color of light yellow, or lemonade, usually indicates adequate hydration.)

- **Evaluate your workout area for falls.** Don't sabotage your safety and success with a dangerous environment. If exercising outside, find an area where the pavement is level and free of cracks. Be aware of curbs, holes in lawns, and the location of driveways; make sure you can cross the street before the light changes. If you plan to exercise indoors, find a room big enough for activity, and remove small carpets and electrical cords from the area.

To avoid injuries, the American Academy of Orthopaedic Surgeons recommends for folks over fifty:[9]

- Warm up with an activity such as brisk walking before you work out to warm up your muscles and get the circulatory system moving; stretch afterwards. Warming up increases your heart and blood flow rates and loosens up muscles and connective tissues.

- Exercise consistently—Aim for thirty minutes of activity on most days of the week, not just on the weekends.

- Use proper equipment—New shoes for walking, helmets for bike riding, and clothing with fibers that allow sweat to evaporate.

- Drink enough water to prevent dehydration and other heat-related problems. Drink 1 pint of water fifteen minutes before you start exercising and another pint after you cool down. Have a drink of water every twenty minutes or so while you exercise.

- Use the 10 percent rule—Gradually increase your activity level. To prevent overuse injuries, increase in increments of no more than 10 percent per week.

OTHER BEST PRACTICES

More than one time, I've almost talked myself out of exercising. It might be because of a lack of time, a cloudy afternoon, or a sore leg. But every time I've gone out for a walk or trip to the gym, I've always felt better afterward. Echoing this sentiment, the older adults in my exercise classes tell me they feel the best after exercising on days they didn't want to come.

So my first advice is: Never pass up an opportunity to engage in physical activity. It *will* lift your mood. Go out and garden—squatting helps strengthen leg muscles and you'll get a good dose of Vitamin D, which many of us lack in our older years. Ride your bike—also good for leg muscles; it will support heart health. Walk your dog—he can become your best personal trainer, reminding you to get outside every day to promote reduced blood pressure, improve your immune system, and lose weight; plus, it's an easy way to meet new people!

Find other activities you enjoy, and start by partaking in them for ten-minute intervals. Then increase the number of days you exercise, as I mentioned above. Aim for three times per day on most days of the week, striving for 150 minutes per week. To boost your chances of success, plan physical activity on your calendar or commit to exercising with a buddy.

When you build up to it, and with your doctor's approval, exercise until your heart beats fast and you work up a sweat. Then you'll begin to enjoy what I call the "afterglow of exercise." This phenomenon is officially known as EPOC (excess post-exercise oxygen consumption). Very simply put, when we exercise, we consume more oxygen and produce energy and chemical by-products. At the same time, we increase breathing, blood circulation, and body temperature above pre-activity levels.

As a result, our metabolism remains high for several minutes to several hours after the exercise bout, resulting in EPOC—the added calories that accompany this post-exercise increase in metabolism. You'll enjoy calorie burning, even when you're not exercising.

EXERCISE

List five ways you'll reach 150 minutes of exercise per week. Include all cardio activities and write them in your calendar.

_____

_____

_____

_____

_____

_____

_____

HIIT THE ROAD

And finally, as your physical condition improves, and again, you have a doctor's okay, experiment with HIIT (high-intensity interval training). HIIT can take care of one of the most common reasons people have for not exercising—a lack of time. It's a super-efficient way to get in shape—a physical activity technique that combines short bouts of nearly all-out effort with periods of recovery. A complete HIIT session takes only 15-20 minutes, and it produces as much (or more) benefit as a sixty-minute moderate-intensity walk.

HIIT can be used with many exercise modalities (walking, bicycling, swimming); it adds variety to your exercise routine and can be used by trained athletes as well as beginners. But here's the best motivation: HIIT allows you to work smarter, not harder, to reap a bucketful of results in a short time.

According to the American College of Sports Medicine,[10] health benefits of HIIT include:

- improved aerobic and anaerobic fitness
- better blood pressure control
- improved cardiovascular health
- improved insulin sensitivity (muscles more readily use glu-

cose for energy)

- better cholesterol profiles

- less abdominal fat and fat just under the skin

- more muscle mass

- reversed age-related muscle decline

HIIT creates a significant amount of stress on the muscles, re-sulting in elevated levels of hormones that increase muscle size. The system trains the body to better tolerate and recover from high-intensity physical activity, and it allows the body to optimally use and store blood sugar, reducing the risk of diabetes.

Before starting a HIIT program, *be sure to be medically cleared.* Then try this beginning version:

- Warm up with 3-5 minutes of comfortable walking.

- Begin your interval: Walk as quickly as possible for fifteen seconds; then slow way down for a minute. (If you think of exercise intensity on a scale of 1-10, with 10 being the most effort you could possibly exert, the "quick" session here should be at least an 8.)

- Repeat five times.

- Cool down with 3-5 minutes of slow walking.

Experiment to determine what works best for your fitness level and goals. You can increase the amount of time you spend in the "high intensity" mode, or increase to 8-10 repetitions. But always include a rest period at least as long as the high-intensity portion. Because of the vigorous effect of HIIT, it's important to limit these sessions to twice a week and allow at least forty-eight hours between.

SUMMARY

To live the life you want well into your later years, cardio is a must. It not only helps decrease the risk and severity of chronic disease, it also supports a healthy brain. No medicine can duplicate all the benefits of exercise!

The good news is many ways exist to reach the cardiovascular, or aerobic, goal of 150 minutes per week. It's not just the organized thirty-minute walk, but everyday activities, such as gardening and housework, that add up. Just find a way to get your big muscles moving for at least ten minutes at a time that allows you to start breathing hard.

Sounds simple, but so many of us don't move enough, for a number of reasons. So how can we motivate ourselves to get regular exercise? One answer: Concentrate on the feeling, as I mentioned in a previous chapter. How do you *feel* during and after exercise? What's the immediate reward, not the long-term health benefits? Once you identify these positive emotions, you have a better chance of continuing with the activity. So pay attention. You might feel more energized right after walking. You might enjoy a sense of accomplishment. You may revel in the sun on your face and wind through your hair while bike riding, or you may relish the feeling of belonging when you work out with others.

Start moving today. Keep moving tomorrow. Begin slowly and safely, and gradually add time and intensity to your exercise program. Like most of my clients and class participants, if you keep it up, cardio won't feel like a chore, but more like a healthy addiction you'll eagerly anticipate on a regular basis.

CHAPTER 10

BUILDING UP YOUR DEFENSES AGAINST CHRONIC DISEASES

PART 1: HEART DISEASE AND DIABETES

"Yes, hello, I'd like a refund on my body.
It's kinda defective and really expensive."

— Anybody with a chronic disease

If you're concentrating on a plant-based diet, moving throughout the day, lifting weights, and getting cardio in your life, you're well on your way to a stronger, healthier future. But you may be worried about how to manage a specific disease. After all, as I quoted earlier in the book, approximately 92 percent of older adults have at least one chronic disease, and 77 percent have two or more.[1]

And Baby Boomers aren't doing much better. Even though we're living longer than our parents, we're more likely to be obese, have diabetes, or have high blood pressure.[2]

In this chapter, I'll take a look at two of the major chronic diseases we're facing in this country: cardiovascular (heart) disease and diabetes. And because full books have been written on them, I'll focus just on factors that are within your control, and how they're related to diet and activity.

Note: All chronic diseases are complex, and it's possible that people can follow all the appropriate recommendations and still have problems. This discussion is not intended to take the place of medical advice.

TAME THE FLAME WITHIN

But first here's a related discussion. One of the gals from my older adult exercise class last year came in with a burning question: What is CRP, and what can I do about it? She'd recently had blood work done and been told her CRP (C-reactive protein) level was high. She thought this was something bad, but she had no idea what to do about it.

CRP, it turns out, provides one assessment of inflammation in the body. This marker has become a measurement regularly included in many routine blood tests. Is chronic inflammation a concern of yours? Here's how CRP can be important to you.

In the past twenty years, researchers have started piecing together a puzzle that connects seemingly unrelated diseases. And amazingly, they're finding just a single culprit, one that can burst plaques, mutate cells, make insulin less efficient, and damage brain cells—it's called chronic inflammation.

Inflammation is our body's defensive response to infection or injury—it's how we limit damage, ward off invading forces, and restore natural balance. When the body senses an injury, it sends out chemicals to activate the immune system. Special cells attack the invader, causing an inflammation that subsides when the danger is over. (Think about a cut on your finger that gets red and swollen, may be hot to touch, and then heals after a few days.)

But when these beneficial processes don't turn off, chronic inflammation follows, attacking healthy cells. This condition is now connected with most chronic diseases, including heart disease, stroke, cancer, depression, and Alzheimer's. Inflammation is also associated with many autoimmune diseases such as celiac and Crohn's disease and rheumatoid arthritis.

While researchers are still unraveling the workings of chronic inflammation, they have put together many suggestions to tame this internal flame. The following are steps you can take to keep inflammation at bay. (Some of these steps I've already discussed while others will be explored in more detail in subsequent chapters.)

1. Stay properly hydrated.
2. Get enough sleep (7-8 hours per night).
3. Increase these:

    - Fruit and vegetables
    - Green tea
    - Omega-3 fatty acids and healthy oils (salmon and tuna, avocados, nuts, seeds, and olive oil)
    - Curcumin—the yellow pigment from the spice, turmeric, has anti-inflammatory properties
    - Homemade meals

4. Decrease these:
    - Sugar intake

- Fatty meat/meat products
- Processed foods

5. Control body weight.

6. Boost your intake of soluble and insoluble fiber (oatmeal, vegetables, nuts, fruits, legumes, seeds, and whole grains).

7. Engage in physical activity, low-to-moderate exercise.

Is your blood work showing signs of inflammation? The next time you go in for a medical checkup, chat with your healthcare provider about this issue.

EXERCISE

List ten ways you can control chronic inflammation. Include food and non-food options.

1. _____

2. _____

3. _____

4. _____

5. _____

6. _____

7. _____

8. _____

9. _____

10. _____

STILL NUMBER ONE! HEART DISEASE

Last year, one of my neighbors shared with me his brush with death, and it mirrors the stories I've heard from other heart-disease patients. In his late fifties, Dave's doctors discovered his arteries were 99 percent blocked; eventually, seven stints would help keep them open. Assuming everything was "fixed," Dave went about his daily life without making any lifestyle changes, but the disease continued to progress.

The real wake-up call didn't occur for another seven years, when a "bad cold"—a side note to a routine doctor's visit—turned out to be a heart attack that led to triple bypass surgery. Dave and his wife have since made major changes to their diet, and he continues to be active in the family business, while enjoying time with his grandchildren.

We all know about heart disease (or cardiovascular disease). Yet despite years of public health efforts to curb this epidemic, the statistics remain alarming:[3]

• Heart disease is still the number-one killer worldwide

• It claims 800,000 US lives each year—approximately one in three deaths

• In the United States, someone dies from a heart attack every forty seconds

"Heart disease" is a category of disorders involving the heart and blood vessels (coronary heart disease, or CHD, and stroke). CHD develops over time, with a narrowing or blockage of heart blood vessels caused by a build-up of plaque (fat and cholesterol). Think of muck gradually accumulating inside a hose, and eventually bursting and blocking the flow of water. This is what happens to blood vessels leading to the heart—eventually they don't allow enough oxygen-rich blood to nourish this vital organ. The result can be a heart attack.

Several risk factors exist for heart disease. Those you *cannot modify* include:

- age (the majority of people who die from heart disease are 65 and older)
- gender (men still have a greater risk of heart disease than women)
- genetics (a family history of heart disease increases the risk, as does being African American, Mexican American, American Indian, or Native Hawaiian)

Fortunately, some *risk factors can be controlled*. The American Heart Association has identified lifestyle goals that contribute to heart health—"Life's Simple 7"[4]—reflected in the recommendations below, divided into Food, Exercise, and Other categories.

Food

1. **Eat better.** Increase your consumption of foods containing soluble fiber, which helps lower cholesterol: fruits (bananas, apples, oranges, peaches, and berries), vegetables (Brussel sprouts and turnips), whole grains (oatmeal), and dried beans. Eat more healthy fats (nuts, seeds, avocado, olive oil) and fish, while cutting down on sodium (salt), overall fat intake (especially saturated and trans fats), high-fat meats (including processed/cured meats), high-fat dairy products, and sugar. These food modifications will help control the following four risk factors.

2. **Control cholesterol.** Cholesterol is a natural substance our bodies manufacture that's vital for its proper functioning. But high levels of one type of cholesterol, LDL, can clog arteries and lead to a heart attack. Diet and exercise affect LDL levels.

3. **Manage blood pressure.** High blood pressure causes excess strain and damage to coronary arteries, which can lead to a build up of plaque and, eventually, a heart attack.

4. **Reduce blood sugar.** Heart disease death rates among adults with diabetes are two to four times higher than adults without diabetes.

5. **Maintain a healthy weight.** A decrease in weight of only 5-10 percent will decrease your overall risk for heart disease.

Physical Activity

6. **Get active.** Exercising thirty minutes most days of the week will boost heart-health.

Other

7. **Stop smoking**—Chemicals in smoke can damage heart tissue and blood vessels. When you quit smoking, your risk of heart disease approximates that of non-smokers within five years.

Also, ask your healthcare provider about plant stanols and sterols, naturally-occurring substances in a plant-based diet that help lower "bad" cholesterol (LDL).

100 MILLION STRONG AND COUNTING: DIABETES

Back in the 1970s, I was a dietetic intern at Miami Valley Hospital in Dayton, Ohio. As I mentioned earlier in the book, part of my education included attending medical lectures at the facility. Some of these meetings stood out so much that I still remember their messages. One of these involved an endocrinologist who was speaking about diabetes, and she made a dire prediction. She said that if Americans didn't start making some big changes, one third of the US population would have diabetes by the year 2030. That number, she said, would cripple the healthcare system and the economy.

Unfortunately, as I've worked in the fitness field, I've seen more and more overweight adults develop this disease.

In fact, more than *30 million Americans now have diabetes*, 9 percent of the population.[5] And that number is more than 400 million worldwide.[6] Even more ominous, another *84 million people*, one in three American adults, have prediabetes. Most of these folks don't even know it, and a good portion of them will go on to have full-blown diabetes within five years if they don't take care of themselves.

And, adding to this problem even further, a recent survey revealed that many primary care physicians may miss a diagnosis of prediabetes because they can't identify risk factors and guidelines for diagnosis.[7]

Diabetes is a group of diseases marked by high levels of blood glucose resulting from defects in insulin production, insulin action, or both. It is the seventh leading cause of death in our country.

Having diabetes *increases the chance for heart disease, stroke, blindness, kidney problems, and nerve damage*. The brain is also at risk—many people with *dementia and Alzheimer's disease* also have diabetes. And the overall risk for death among some groups of people with diabetes is higher than that of those without the disease.[8]

The major types of diabetes are:

* Type 1 diabetes, in which the body does not produce enough insulin to convert food into energy, is usually diagnosed in children.

These people must take insulin daily.

- In type 2 diabetes (T2), the most common form of diabetes, the body doesn't use insulin efficiently ("insulin resistance"). Although the pancreas tries to keep up with demand, eventually it is unable to make enough of the hormone to keep blood sugar levels normal. As the incidence of obesity has risen, so has the prevalence of type 2 diabetes. Thus, folks with T2 control the disease with diet, exercise, weight loss, and oral medications. (Sometimes insulin is required.)

- Gestational diabetes develops during pregnancy. Although the high blood sugar levels can affect both mother and baby's health, they usually return to normal after delivery.

And while most experts believe type 2 diabetes is not reversible, it is possible to stop prediabetes from becoming T2. In fact, thousands of people with prediabetes participated in a national study, the Diabetes Prevention Program, and reduced their chances of developing diabetes by 58 percent through lifestyle changes.[9]

Here are strategies to help better control your blood sugar, from the American Diabetes Association (ADA)[10]:

Food

ADA recognizes a variety of food patterns to control prediabetes and T2, including the Mediterranean, DASH (Dietary Approaches to Stop Hypertension), and plant-based diets.

- *Manage your weight.* A loss of just 5-7 percent of initial weight improves blood sugar control and reduces the need for glucose-lowering medications.

- *Decrease caloric intake by 500-750 calories per day* for modest weight loss.

- *Emphasize fruits and vegetables, whole grain products, and legumes.* The fiber in these foods takes more time to digest, helps you feel full longer, and controls spikes in blood sugar.

- *Include nuts and seeds and moderate amounts of low-fat dairy and lean meats.*

Physical Activity

During exercise, muscle contractions increase the use of glucose for energy, lowering blood sugar levels for several hours. Both resistance training and aerobic exercise improve blood glucose control.

ADA recommends people with diabetes:

- *Decrease sedentary behavior*; interrupt prolonged sitting every thirty minutes.

- Get at least *150 minutes of moderate-to-vigorous exercise per week* spread over at least three days/week, with no more than two consecutive days without activity.

- *Engage in strength-training activities* two to three times per week on non-consecutive days.

- *Participate in flexibility and balance training* two to three times per week.

Other

- *Know your numbers.* Ask your doctor to check your fasting blood sugar (FBS). The ideal level is less than 100. Doctors also use the A1C test, which reflects a person's average blood glucose levels over the past three months without daily fluctuations.

  o An FBS level of 100 - 125, or A1C level of 5.7 to 6.4, indicates prediabetes.

- o   An FBS level of 126 or above, or A1C level of 6.5 or above, is diabetes.

- *Manage stress and depression*, which can raise one's risk of diabetes.

EXERCISE

If you have, or are concerned about getting, heart disease or diabetes, write five food changes and five physical activity changes you can make to help better control your health.

Food Changes	Physical Activity Changes
_____	_____
_____	_____
_____	_____
_____	_____
_____	_____

SUMMARY

Six of the seven leading causes of death are chronic diseases. Most experts now agree these are *not* a normal part of aging, and they can be managed with appropriate changes in lifestyle.

In this chapter, we discussed two of these disorders: heart disease and diabetes. In both cases, diet and physical activity play key roles in controlling or reversing the conditions by managing blood sugar, "bad" cholesterol levels, blood pressure, and body weight.

The key food components to defend against these chronic diseases are a plant-based, Mediterranean, or DASH diet, that includes:

- fruits, vegetables, legumes (dried peas and beans), and whole-grain products
- healthy fats from nuts, seeds, olives/olive oil, avocados, and fatty fish
- some researchers recommend including foods high in potassium to help guard against diseases of the heart and circulatory system (sweet and white potatoes, winter squash, white beans, yogurt, oranges, bananas)
- foods with magnesium may help protect against diabetes (spinach, chard, pumpkin seeds, yogurt, almonds, black beans, avocados, dark chocolate)

Best practices for physical activity include:

- 150 minutes of challenging and consistent moderate-to-vigorous cardiovascular or aerobic exercise per week (for example, thirty minutes on most days of the week) or seventy-five minutes of vigorous activity
- increasing movement throughout the day by breaking up sedentary activity every 30-60 minutes
- strength or resistance training at least twice a week on non-consecutive days
- flexibility and balance training at least twice a week

Individuals should always check with their healthcare professionals before starting a new eating pattern or exercise program, es-

pecially older adults with chronic diseases controlled by medications.

But the good news is that small changes can lead to big gains in wellness. For example, even a moderate weight loss of 5-10 percent in total body weight results in improved blood pressure, blood cholesterol, and blood sugar. This should encourage you to start changing your lifestyle, no matter your age, to live a longer, stronger, more vibrant life.

CHAPTER 11

BUILDING UP YOUR DEFENSES AGAINST CHRONIC DISEASES

Part 2: CANCER AND DEMENTIA/ALZHEIMER'S

"Cancer didn't bring me to my knees;
it brought me to my feet."

— Michael Douglas

In Chapter 10, we started our discussion of chronic diseases with a candid look at heart disease and diabetes. These two conditions share several risk factors and lifestyle prevention/treatment strategies. In this chapter, I'll move on to cancer and dementia/ Alzheimer's disease. These two disease classifications top the list of conditions that frighten most Americans. What we'll learn is that only a small amount of risk for these diseases is destined through your genes; diet and exercise (along with other factors) greatly increase or decrease the odds.

Note: All chronic diseases are complex, and it's possible that people can follow all the appropriate recommendations and still have problems. This discussion is not intended to take the place of medical advice.

THE SCARY "C" WORD—CANCER

I can still remember the phone call from my mother. It was early September, 1987, and I was pregnant with our second daughter. My parents had recently returned from an overseas vacation, and my dad had been experiencing marked shortness of breath. The first word we'd gotten from the doctors was fluid in the lungs. But this phone call held the diagnosis that turned my world upside down: incurable lung cancer.

The doctors gave my father eighteen months to live. During that time, our new daughter and nephew were born, my parents celebrated their fortieth wedding anniversary, and my father lost a great deal of weight as the cancer ate away at him. He died at home just after Christmas 1988. The threat of cancer has haunted our family ever since.

Cancer is a disease in which cells act abnormally. That is, rather than dividing and dying off when they become old or damaged, cancer cells begin to divide without stopping and spread into surrounding tissues.

More than 100 types of cancer exist. The most common are breast cancer, lung and bronchus cancer, prostate cancer, colon and rectum cancer, bladder cancer, melanoma of the skin, non-Hodgkin lymphoma, thyroid cancer, kidney and renal pelvis cancer, leukemia, endometrial cancer, and pancreatic cancer.[1]

Cancer is a genetic disease because we can inherit genetic tendencies from our parents (thus my and my kids' fear of cancer). And DNA can be damaged from environmental "attacks" such as tobacco smoke, radiation, or ultraviolet rays from the sun.

But experts agree that *only 5-10 percent of all cancers are due to inherited mutations.*[2]

And while researchers cannot pinpoint the causes of all cancers, *advancing age* is the most important risk factor, with the median age of cancer diagnosis at age sixty-six.[3]

Having said that, many other risk factors can be controlled to decrease your risk of developing cancer.[4]

(NOTE: Because there are so many different types of cancer, check with your own physician to pinpoint lifestyle changes that work best for your case.)

Food

For the most part, you control what you eat. Take advantage of that reality.

- *Eat a variety of whole foods, and do not depend on dietary supplements.* According to the American Cancer Society, "research does not support their use in lowering cancer risk."
- *Eat a variety of fruits and vegetables*, at least 2½ cups per day. I've mentioned previously that diets with a higher vegetable and fruit intake reduce cancer risk.
- *Choose whole-grain breads, pasta, and cereals.*
- *Limit your intake of refined carbohydrate foods and high-sugar foods.*
- *Limit high-fat foods.*

- *Limit red and processed meats.* The World Health Organization has concluded there is "sufficient evidence from epidemiological studies that eating processed meat causes colorectal cancer."[5]
- Prepare meat, poultry, and fish by *baking, broiling, or poaching rather than by frying or charbroiling.*
- *Control body weight and avoid obesity.* Absence of excess body fat lowers the risk of most cancers.[6]

Physical Activity

I may be sounding like a broken record, but *movement* is critical in avoiding chronic diseases, including cancer.

- *Physical activity decreases the risk of cancers* of the breast, colon, endometrium, and prostate, and possibly others.
- Find a physical activity you enjoy, and aim for *150 minutes weekly.*
- *Limit sedentary behavior* (sitting, lying down, watching television, or other forms of screen-based entertainment).

Other

- *Limit alcohol intake* to no more than two drinks per day for men and one drink per day for women. Alcohol has been linked to the increased risk of several cancers, including those of the mouth, esophagus, liver, breast, and colon/rectum.
- *Do not smoke.* Smoking accounts for about 30 percent of all cancer deaths in the United States; it damages airways and cells in the lungs.
- *Limit sun exposure.* Ultraviolet (UV) light causes skin cancer; limit exposure to it between 10:00 a.m. and 4:00 p.m. by stay-

ing out of the sun, using protective clothing, and applying sunscreen.

YOUR BRAIN—YOU CAN HELP IT STAY YOUNG

When I talk with Baby Boomers, one of their biggest fears is Alzheimer's disease (AD). This is especially worrisome for folks whose parents suffer from dementia. I understand this—there's no definitive cause and no known cure for AD. And the mental decline and personality changes are a scary future to envision.

In my area of Southern California, I have noticed several new memory care facilities going up in recent years. At a local networking meeting, I had the opportunity to tour one of these facilities. While administrators are trying hard to create a "homey" environment for clients and provide clues to spur memories from clients' pasts (for example, military experience and marriage), the locked doors and limited access are constant reminders of the occurring ravages of the mind.

So let's take a quick look at dementia and AD; then we'll focus on lifestyle factors that might help you avoid these diseases.

As we grow older, our brains go through natural changes that result in subtle declines in mental function: we can't process information as quickly, we don't "multitask" as well, and parts of our memory start to decline, as does our ability to make decisions. But none of these changes affect our ability to function in everyday life.

With dementia, a greater deterioration happens in memory, thinking, behavior, and the ability to perform everyday activities; this is *not a normal part of growing older*.

AD is the most common form of dementia. In fact, 60 percent of folks who suffer from dementia have AD. AD leads to personality changes and slowly destroys brain health, with declines in memory and thinking skills, and eventually, the ability to carry out the simplest tasks of daily life.

Consider these statistics from the Alzheimer's Organization: More than 5 million Americans have AD; every sixty seconds, someone in the United States develops AD; one in three seniors dies with AD or another dementia; AD kills more than breast and prostate cancer combined; dementia is the most expensive disease in the United States; and by the year 2050, triple the number of people will be living with AD. The greatest risk factor for the disease is increasing age.[7]

Clearly, the need to find preventive strategies is critical. Luckily, researchers are making some progress. For example, many of the folks suffering from AD also have obesity, type 2 diabetes, and hypertension—chronic diseases that respond to lifestyle changes. Let's take a look at some recent recommendations.

Food

One of the theories of aging goes like this: With increasing age, our bodies often don't react as well to everyday stress and illness. Cells can be damaged by "free radicals," molecules that are normally taken care of by our natural antioxidants. But when these molecules overwhelm this defense system, they can cause chronic inflammation and diseases such as Alzheimer's.

So researchers are looking at food patterns that help squelch this process with antioxidants and anti-inflammatories. Both the Mediterranean diet and DASH diet (originally developed to treat high blood pressure) fit the bill and have been associated with cardiovascular and brain protection. They also promote mental health by increasing blood flow to the brain, bringing in oxygen and needed nutrients, and taking out waste products.

Both diets are high in fruits and vegetables, whole grains, healthy fats, and legumes and nuts, with some lean protein sources. They are low in sugar and harmful fats.

Researchers at Rush University Medical Center took the best parts of these programs and developed the MIND diet.[8] Their results: The risk of AD was lowered by as much as 53 percent in participants who adhered to the diet rigorously (the equivalent of their brain function being 7.5 years younger).

Here are some *best practices* from the three diets mentioned above:

1. Ensure the majority of your diet consists of:

- fruits and vegetables, up to 11 servings per day, stressing berries and green leafy vegetables
- dried beans about 3-4 times per week
- whole grains, at least 3 serving per day
- olive oil
- nuts
- a small amount of fish and poultry, once or twice a week
- wine, in small amounts

2. Limit:

- red meats
- pastries and sweets
- fried or fast food
- fats from meat sources

Physical Activity

Many of my clients and class participants know that moving just makes them feel better. They attribute these benefits to the increase in endorphins, our feel-good chemicals. But physical activity's benefits go even deeper, changing the brain's actual structure to support healthy aging.

Aging leads to a decrease of blood, oxygen, and nutrients to the brain, and a drop in the number of brain cells (neurons) and all-important connections between them (synapses). Simply put, the stresses of everyday living can cause neurons and synapses to decay, possibly leading to brain dysfunction or dementias.

Scientists once thought we were born with a finite number of brain cells; when they died off, they were gone, along with the functions they performed. It was believed nothing could be done to reverse this process.

But researchers now know we're capable of rebuilding our brains through a process called "neuroplasticity." The brain is actually capable of rewiring its circuits, bringing back the ability to adapt to new circumstances and develop new skills.

This is where exercise comes in—hailed as one of the most promising lifestyle interventions for the prevention of several brain maladies, including Alzheimer's. Exercise increases blood flow to the brain and helps control many of AD's co-morbidities: diabetes, cardiovascular disease, and obesity.

But most importantly, it turns out that *physical activity*, especially aerobic or cardiovascular exercise, *promotes the production of special proteins called brain-derived neurotropic factors* (BDNF), as I mentioned in a previous chapter. These chemicals stimulate new connections between brain cells, generate new blood vessels, and produce new brain cells. And again, because it ushers in neuroplasticity, BDNF has been likened to "Miracle Grow for our brains."[9]

BDNF helps protect our brains. A 2016 study of 533 older adults found that those with higher levels of BDNF had slower rates of mental decline.[10]

While all exercise (both strength training and cardio) increases the synthesis of BDNF, the "secret sauce" may be combining aerobic exercise with complex physical activities that are mentally stimulating, engaging, and skill-based. Some examples might include throwing a ball back and forth while walking, reciting the alphabet backwards while using the elliptical, or even (safe) rock climbing. The key is to keep your brain challenged. Even changing up your workout or trying new routines will help.

Here's the bottom line with exercise for robust brain health:

- Twice weekly, engage in strength training.
- Weekly, include 150 minutes of consistent and mentally challenging aerobic exercise.
- Twice weekly, work on balance and flexibility training to prevent falls because head injuries are a major risk factor for Alzheimer's disease.

ADDENDUM

As I was completing work on this chapter, some important findings were released.[11] At the 2017 Alzheimer's Association International Conference in London, experts concluded that *one third of the world's cases of dementia could be prevented by targeting the following nine risk factors.* (By comparison, these experts stated targeting the major *genetic* aspect of dementia would prevent only 7 percent of cases):

- staying in school until at least age fifteen
- reducing hearing loss

- avoiding obesity between ages 45-65
- avoiding high blood pressure between ages 45-65
- reducing smoking
- reducing depression
- reducing physical inactivity
- reducing social isolation
- avoiding diabetes after age sixty-five

Additional recommendations from these experts include: avoid heart disease, get 7-8 hours of sleep per night, avoid head injuries, and drink moderately, if at all.

Is developing AD a concern of yours? What about cancer? Are you ready to help boost your defenses against these debilitating diseases?

EXERCISE

Depending on the chronic disease most pertinent to you, write five food changes and five physical activity changes you can make to better help control your health.

Food Changes	Physical Activity Changes

SUMMARY

This chapter tackled two major classes of chronic disease: cancers and dementias/Alzheimer's disease. Together, cancers and dementias/AD cost the nation almost $400 billion annually, and those numbers are expected to continue rising.[12]

Cancer is the second leading cause of death in our country; Alzheimer's disease is number six. More than 47 million people worldwide have dementia; most of them suffer with AD.[13]

In the case of cancers and AD, cells in the body become abnormal and out of control. Diseases develop over many years. But it's critical to remember that less than 10 percent of your risk for developing these diseases is inherited; modifiable factors play a much larger role in decreasing your risk of developing them.

Eating guidelines for these conditions include:

- Eat a variety of whole foods, especially fruits and vegetables.
- Choose whole-grain breads, pasta, and cereals while limiting highly processed carbohydrates and high-sugar foods. Spices add flavor and antioxidant and anti-inflammatory properties.
- Limit high-fat meats, especially red meats and processed/cured meats.
- Control body weight and avoid obesity.

Activity recommendations include:

- 150 minutes per week of cardiovascular exercise that you enjoy doing.
- Mentally and physically challenging activities, done consistently.
- Limiting sedentary behavior.
- Strength training, flexibility, and balance training two days per week.

Individuals should always check with their healthcare professionals before starting a new eating pattern or exercise program, espe-

cially older adults with chronic diseases controlled by medications.

So don't sit around waiting to see what Mother Nature has in store for you, especially if you have one of these conditions in your family tree. Take advantage of that majority of risk that you can control, and get started today living a healthier life tomorrow.

CHAPTER 12

BUILDING UP YOUR DEFENSES AGAINST CHRONIC DISEASES

Part 3: ARTHRITIS AND OSTEOPOROSIS

"The way I deal with arthritis is to keep moving....
As long as you can, do it...."

— Robert Redford

In the previous chapters, we discussed choices you can make to help manage heart disease, diabetes, cancer, and dementia/ Alzheimer's. In this chapter, we'll tackle the debilitating conditions that take aim at the body's structural framework—joints and bones: arthritis and osteoporosis.

Taken together, these diseases afflict more than 90 million Americans, many of them Baby Boomers and older adults.[1] Worldwide, arthritis and related disorders represent one of the highest causes of disability. And osteoporosis leads to more than 8.9 million fractures per year.[2]

Similar to guidelines in Chapters 10 and 11, what you eat and how you move can impact your odds of developing and managing these conditions.

Note: All chronic diseases are complex, and it's possible that people can follow all the appropriate recommendations and still have problems. This discussion is not intended to take the place of medical advice.

A CRIPPLING DISEASE—ARTHRITIS

Does arthritis "run" in your family? As long as I can remember, my mother was fighting joint disease. The first signs of arthritis were in her hands—swollen joints and bent fingers. Later in life, she suffered from hip arthritis and would go on to have hip, shoulder, and knee replacements due to this disabling disease, which limited her ability to live an independent life.

Unfortunately, arthritis seems to "run" in our family—I'm currently dealing with severe bone-on-bone arthritis in my left hip, and a replacement surgery is in my future also.

According to the Arthritis Foundation,[3] one in four adults, or nearly 54 million people, have doctor-diagnosed arthritis. Arthritis includes more than 100 rheumatic diseases and conditions that affect joints, the tissues that surround the joint and other connective tissue. The most common type of arthritis is osteoarthritis. Its main symptoms are joint pain, swelling, and stiffness; these usually grow worse with age, although the CDC states arthritis is "not a normal part of aging."[4] (It's considered a "wear and tear" disease.)

Scientists don't know exactly what causes or how to prevent arthritis, and it's generally considered incurable. Being female and having a family history of the disorder increases your risk of developing arthritis. But other risk factors are modifiable.

Food

For osteoarthritis, *maintain a healthy weight*. Extra pounds put additional loads on joints and limit mobility. They also make recovery from joint replacement surgery more difficult and put stress on new prosthetic components.

Much has been written about foods to eat or avoid for arthritis care, but the consensus seems to be to consume a *Mediterranean-type diet:* 3-4 ounces of fish twice a week, nuts and seeds, fruits and vegetables (berries, cherries, spinach, kale, and broccoli), olive oil, and whole grains.[5]

These foods are filling and full of beneficial phytochemicals, antioxidants, and anti-inflammatories.

Some people with arthritis avoid *nightshade vegetables* (eggplant, tomatoes, potatoes, and red bell peppers). Although there's no scientific evidence that this practice helps relieve arthritic pain, if you believe they're affecting your arthritis, try eliminating all nightshade veggies for a few weeks to see whether you notice a difference.

Others find *glucosamine* helpful, but according to the National Center for Complementary and Integrative Health, studies have produced conflicting evidence about whether the supplement reduces joint pain.[6] Check with your doctor before trying out these supplements because they can interfere with the blood thinner Coumadin and may affect your body's ability to handle blood sugar.

Physical Activity

A natural reaction to arthritis is to curtail movement. I know because it's happening to me with my hip pain, so I've switched from walking to swimming and bicycling. But the results of inactivity can be catastrophic, as I've discussed in other chapters, leading to a downward spiral toward permanent disability.

So movement is imperative; my physical therapist likes to say, "Motion is the lotion!" Exercise encourages the circulation of synovial fluid, which lubricates joints; it increases blood flow to pump oxygen and nutrients to affected areas, and it helps remove wastes.

Work with your healthcare providers to design an individualized program for your specific arthritis needs. Engage in *strength training twice a week* to improve muscle strength around the affected joint, resulting in less stress on the joint, reduced pain and joint stiffness, and improved maintenance of functional abilities.

Strive for *150 minutes of cardio per week*, following the guidelines in the previous chapter. Start slowly, noting which activities your body tolerates. Be sure to include plenty of time to warm up (heat relaxes muscles and increases circulation); then find aerobic exercises you enjoy that do not twist or pound your joints.

Excellent examples include *walking, swimming, and water-based exercises, stationary biking*, and *yoga*. Applying ice after exercise can help decrease pain and inflammation. Check with the Arthritis Foundation or your local YMCA for programs in your area.

And don't forget flexibility and balance exercises, which I'll discuss in the chapter about fall prevention.

Are you battling arthritis, so you're starting to cut back on exercise from fear of exacerbating the pain?

EXERCISE

If you have arthritis, use the columns below to come up with a plan to manage it. On the left-hand side, list the activities you've limited because of your condition. These may be stair climbing, brisk walking, or household chores. Be honest with yourself.

Now, on the right-hand side, list three ways you can help control the disease. It may be weight loss, exercise (be specific), or improving your diet with more fruits and vegetables and less sugar and harmful fats. The more specific you can get, the better the chances you can make these happen.

Activities	Ways to Control the Disease

THEM BONES, THEM BONES!—OSTEOPOROSIS

Although I don't need the reminder, my clients frequently tease me with the following statement, "It comes with the territory!" They're talking, of course, about their chronic diseases, which constantly challenge me to come up with Plans B, C, and maybe even D when it comes to strength-training exercises.

169

For example, twice weekly I have the privilege of leading an exercise class for older adults. And I mean older—folks in their seventies and eighties. Before participants enter the program, we screen on paper for chronic diseases, and one of the issues I often see is osteoporosis. Depending on which part(s) of the body is affected, I modify the exercises so they're safe for everyone, like Jane, who has osteoporosis in her back. We are very careful not to have her bend or twist at the waist to protect her spine.

According to the National Osteoporosis Foundation, about 54 million Americans have osteoporosis and low bone mass.[7] Osteoporosis is a condition characterized by low bone density, resulting in brittle and weak bones. (Osteopenia is a term referring to low bone density, but not low enough to be classified as osteoporosis.)

You may not be aware of it, but our bones are not static, unchanging structures; they're constantly "on the move." During childhood and adolescence, we're building and breaking down bones all the time, storing minerals such as calcium, phosphorus, and magnesium in our skeletons.

But after age thirty, we begin to lose more bone than we construct. As a result, our bones are less dense or strong, making osteoporosis the leading cause of broken bones in adults over the age of fifty. In fact, approximately one in two women and up to one in four men age fifty and older will break a bone due to this condition.

Like many chronic diseases, osteoporosis develops over a lifetime. Many seniors learn of its existence only after breaking a bone. And, validating that key worry my mother and her friends had a few years back, falls often lead to broken bones, severely limiting mobility for older adults. Furthermore, 20 percent of seniors who break a hip die within one year, and many others require long-term nursing home care.

A long list of health conditions and medications can lead to bone loss. *So if you're over fifty and have any of the following risk factors, ask your doctor for a full medical review and insist on osteoporosis screening (DEXA is the gold standard screening procedure)*:

- you've broken a bone
- you're female (approximately 80 percent of all osteoporosis cases are in women)
- you have a small frame
- you're on the thin side
- you're Caucasian or Asian

Food

Here are ways food intake can tip the scales in your favor with regards to protecting from bone loss:

1. Consume adequate amounts of *calcium* in the form of foods before turning to supplements. The best absorbed sources of calcium in our diet are *dairy products* (milk, yogurt, and cheese), which are frequently fortified with vitamin D, needed for calcium absorption. Other good sources include:

   - *Leafy greens* (such as kale and collard greens) and broccoli (Note: spinach contains oxalic acid, which binds onto calcium to block its absorption; do not eat with other high calcium foods.)
   - *Canned sardines and salmon* (with bones)

2. Eat a wide *variety of fruits and vegetables* to get other nutrients needed for bone health (potassium, magnesium, vitamins C and K).

3. Ask your doctor to check your *Vitamin D* level; if it's too low, it doesn't matter how much calcium you take in; it won't be absorbed and won't be used.

    *   Sun exposure helps our bodies make Vitamin D.
    *   Dietary sources of vitamin D include: fatty fishes such as salmon, mackerel, tuna, and sardines.
    *   Vitamin D supplementation may be needed; check with your healthcare provider for the amount.

4. Consume *adequate protein* (more in Chapter 15).

Physical Activity

1. Speak to your healthcare professional before starting an exercise program.
2. Work with a physical therapist or personal trainer to be sure the exercises are safe and appropriate.
3. Start slowly and allow 5-10 minutes for warm-up and cooldown (slow movement of joints through range of motion or low-intensity activity).
4. Include *weight-bearing and strength-training exercises* that help keep muscles and bones strong.

    *   For strength-training, use free weights, weight machines, body weight, or resistance tubes or bands.
    *   Weight-bearing exercises include brisk walking, dancing, low-impact aerobics, stair climbing, and elliptical training.

5. *Avoid*:

    *   High-impact exercises such as jumping, running, or jogging
    *   Activities that require bending or twisting at the waist (sit-

ups, golf, bowling; reaching down to pick up items from the floor)

- Jerky, rapid movements

- Solely depending on water-based exercises; these do not strengthen bones

6. Also work on flexibility and balance to avoid falls.

Other

1. Some medications can lead to bone loss. Check with your physician.

2. Some medications that help control bone loss have serious side effects. Again, check with your physician.

3. Limit alcohol to no more than 2-3 drinks per day. (Heavy drinking can lead to bone loss.)

4. Stop smoking.

5. Osteogenic loading is a procedure that applies force to the bones to stimulate their natural ability to increase density.[8] Ask your healthcare provider about programs such as OsteoStrong, that are proven to increase bone density and muscle strength using this principle.

Is bone loss a concern for you now, or possibly in your future?

EXERCISE

If osteoporosis affects you, or if you're worried about developing this condition, write five food and five physical activity changes you can make to help boost your health.

Food Changes	Physical Activity Changes
_____	_____
_____	_____
_____	_____
_____	_____
_____	_____

SUMMARY

In this chapter, we finished our discussion of chronic diseases. Arthritis and osteoporosis are both extremely debilitating diseases, costing millions of dollars and leading to a decline in health for many older adults worldwide.

As with the conditions discussed in Chapters 10 and 11, many risk factors exist for these diseases that we cannot change or avoid. But evidence also exists that positive lifestyle changes can prevent or mitigate the effects of arthritis and osteoporosis. Keep your weight down, concentrate on nutritious fruits, vegetables, and calcium sources, and, as always, find ways to keep moving, even when your brain tells you to sit this one out!

Check with your healthcare provider, dietitian, or physical therapist for the course of treatment that best suits your case. Find solutions that work, and stick with them.

Individuals should always check with their healthcare professionals before starting a new eating pattern or exercise program, es-

pecially older adults with chronic diseases controlled by medications.

(Note: I have not included many medications for the treatment of chronic diseases in my discussions. Again, I urge you to talk with your doctor to determine the best treatment for your particular situation.)

CHAPTER 13

SHEDDING A FEW POUNDS, AND KEEPING THEM OFF

"Losing weight is simple, but it's not easy!"

— Leslie Nardini

In the past three chapters, I've laid out choices we can all make to help avoid or mitigate the negative consequences of chronic diseases. However, one chronic disease I haven't mentioned yet impacts all others: obesity.

In 2013, the American Medical Association officially declared obesity and being overweight to be a "chronic medical disease state." In doing so, the AMA recognized obesity as an urgent public health problem and opened the way for healthcare professionals to start treating the problem seriously as it relates to other chronic diseases.[1]

In this chapter, I'll lay out the case for controlling extra pounds, explore just how much weight loss is needed to help improve your health, and offer best practices for winning the battle of the bulge.

AGAIN, MOTHER NATURE'S NOT HELPING US

Every once in a while, I survey my "peeps" to find out what they're worried about to make sure my services are meeting their needs. Invariably, difficulty in keeping weight off shows up at the top of the list. Is this one of your big worries?

For a number of reasons, this isn't surprising. After all, 70 percent of Boomers are overweight or obese, resulting in an increased risk of diabetes, heart disease, and cancer. Unfortunately, it's not easy to keep weight off with advancing years. In fact, here's how the odds are naturally stacked against us for staying slim as we age:

1. As we grow older, we are usually not as active. This decreases our need for calories.

2. A process called sarcopenia starts to take its toll. (We talked about this in Chapter 8.) From our thirties on, we start to lose muscle mass, also called lean body mass (LBM). In fact, we lose about 3-5 percent per decade. We end up with a proportionately higher percentage of body fat, which brings about increased risk for chronic diseases.

3. Lean muscle burns more calories in a resting state than does fat. So if you have less LBM, your resting metabolism—the rate at which your body burns calories to maintain basic functions—goes down. This decrease is critical because resting metabolism accounts for the majority of all calorie burning throughout the day.

Bottom line: If you continue eating the same number of calories as the years move on without changing your level of activity, you'll gradually gain weight. In fact, the Harvard Medical School reports the average person gains about 3-4 lbs per year starting in middle age.[2]

So we intentionally have to watch our eating and activity to keep weight from creeping up on us.

Has your weight "naturally" increased over the years?

EXERCISE

Note your weight when you got married. Next, for women, where did the scale sit at the conception of your first, second, or third child? Do your pants or skirts from three or four years ago still fit you? For guys, what's happened to your pants size over the years? Record the information below, along with an honest assessment of your weight history from young adulthood until now.

_____

_____

_____

SO WHAT IF I'VE GAINED A FEW POUNDS?

I remember an executive I met while doing my fitness internship. George had let his weight go because he was too busy to exercise. He saw his weight mainly as an inconvenience. (His golf games were getting more difficult.) It wasn't until he was riding in the back of an ambulance that he understood the serious health implications of his lifestyle. And he was one of the lucky ones; not everybody survives a major heart attack.

But most people do understand obesity is more than a cosmetic problem. In fact, it's widely recognized as one of the biggest causes of preventable chronic diseases and high healthcare costs in the country.

Just what is the definition of obesity or being overweight? If you're overweight, you probably know it. But how can you tell if you're obese? Being overweight or obese is primarily measured with a calculation called the BMI, body mass index. The easiest way to determine your BMI is to look at a chart found in most doctors' offices or go online and plug in numbers. Here's one site you can use from the National Institutes of Health: https://www.nhlbi.nih.gov/health/educational/lose_wt/BMI/bmicalc.htm (or just Google BMI).

Other ways exist to measure obesity, and BMI is not accurate for some people (the elderly and heavily muscled individuals). But it's still the accepted standard for determining whether someone is overweight or obese, and for comparing his or her weight to that of other population groups.

- A BMI of 18.5-24.9 is considered normal.
- A BMI of 25-29.9 is considered overweight.
- A BMI of greater than 30 is considered obese.

In the United States, obesity costs range up to $210 billion per year; increasing BMI leads to higher absenteeism, lower productivity at work, and higher medical claims and healthcare costs.[3]

And when it comes to extra weight and chronic disease, researchers cannot always pinpoint an exact cause and effect. But reviews of hundreds of studies can draw an association between obesity and the diseases we discussed in the previous three chapters.

Let's look at some specifics:

Heart disease: 21 percent of chronic heart disease can be attributed to a BMI over 21.[4]

Diabetes: Being overweight or obese is the single best predictor of type 2 diabetes. Nearly 90 percent of people living with type 2 diabetes are overweight or have obesity.[5]

Cancer: Higher amounts of body fat are associated with increased risk of several cancers, including: breast (in post-menopausal women), endometrial, liver, kidney, colorectal, and multiple myeloma.[6]

Brain health: Obesity increases the risk of dementia in general by 42 percent, Alzheimer's by 80 percent.[7]

Arthritis: A five-unit increase in BMI increases the risk of both hip and knee osteoarthritis[8] and[9].

Waist circumference: Measure your waist circumference around the narrowest part of your torso (just above the belly button).

- For men, more than 40" is related to an increase of chronic diseases.
- For women, more than 35" is the cut-off.

As I said, the exact mechanism by which obesity leads to chronic diseases is not known. It could be that obese individuals have more chronic inflammation, higher levels of insulin and related hormones, excess amounts of estrogen, or depressed immune responses. Or it could be that folks who are obese also have high blood pressure and higher "bad" cholesterol levels. Or it could be the complex relationship between the various diseases themselves that are more prevalent in obese individuals.

Whatever the case, it's clear that controlling weight is critical for living a life with minimal chronic disease and maximal functional independence.

A SMALL LOSS = A BIG GAIN

Does this sound familiar? You jump on the scale and tell yourself, "I need to lose a lot of weight!" Maybe it's twenty, forty, or sixty pounds. Whatever the number, most people think in terms of a specific "dream" weight they want to achieve. The problem is that achieving that goal can be overwhelming, and if the ultimate goal isn't met, people get discouraged and stop trying. Then they regain the weight, and the classic yo-yo dieting/weight-gain pattern begins.

But some encouraging news has come up in the last few years regarding how much weight loss leads to improved health. This approach encourages smaller weight loss goals and emphasizes that it's more important to think of losing weight as a way to increase wellness as opposed to thinking about how you look.

- A loss of 5-10 percent of initial weight can lead to an improvement of risk factors for heart disease and diabetes.[10]
- The results of the Diabetes Prevention Program, following more than 3,000 people, showed that those individuals at high risk for developing the disease who lost at least 7 percent of initial weight through lifestyle intervention (diet and physical activity) reduced the risk of developing diabetes by 58 percent.[11]

So it's time to rethink your weight loss goals. If you weigh 200 pounds, a 5 percent loss is 10 pounds. That's where health benefits begin.

Then hold that weight for 6-12 months before trying to lose more weight. Studies show that weight loss and maintenance get easier with time, so be patient. You didn't get to your current weight overnight—you know where I'm going with this!

And take heart from the 10,000 individuals who are being tracked in the National Weight Control Registry.[12] This registry provides information about the strategies used by successful dieters to achieve and maintain long-term weight loss. (Members must have lost at least thirty pounds and kept it off for one year.) After individuals have *successfully maintained their weight loss for 2-5 years, the chance of longer-term success greatly increases.*

EXERCISE

What would be a healthful weight loss goal for you (5-10 percent)? Write down the number below.

_____

BEST PRACTICES FOR WEIGHT LOSS

People are constantly asking me which type of diet is best. Some folks know others who've had tremendous success with low-carb diets; others have tried meal programs like Nutrisystem, while still others love Weight Watchers. So just which program is best for weight loss?

In an attempt to answer that question, researchers evaluated results of forty-eight clinical trials including 7,286 individuals. They compared weight loss at six and twelve months for those on diets versus no diet. Researchers sought to determine weight-loss outcomes for popular diet plans such as Atkins, Zone, Weight Watchers, and Nutrisystem.[13]

The results:

- Compared to no diet, the low-carbohydrate diets had a median difference in weight loss of 19.2 pounds at six months, and 16.0 pounds at twelve months.

- Low-fat diets had a mean difference of 17.6 pounds at six months, and 16.0 pounds at twelve months.

The conclusion: "Significant weight loss was observed with any low-carbohydrate or low-fat diet. Weight loss differences between individual named diets were small. This supports the practice of *recommending any diet that a patient will adhere to in order to lose weight.*" The key is to create a sustained deficit of caloric intake.

Which brings us to the crux of the issue: Weight loss and maintenance is a lifelong journey. Losing weight can't be boiled down to "going on" a diet and then "going off." Dr. Yoni Freedhoff, a Canadian weight-loss expert who has worked with more than 40,000 clients, sums it up perfectly: "If you don't like the life you're living while you're losing weight, you're virtually certain to gain it back."[14] He asks only for your best effort to live the healthiest life possible, eating the least number of calories and exercising the most hours you're comfortable with.

Permanent weight loss results from a lifelong commitment to lifestyle changes. And for a successful program, it's important to understand that most fitness professionals agree: weight loss is 70-80 percent food intake, 20-30 percent exercise. It's just too easy to eat back those 300 calories you've just taken an hour to burn off. (One coffeehouse drink will do it!)

So remember: Lose weight in the kitchen. Gain health in the gym!

In summary, here are eleven strategies for successful weight loss and maintenance:

1. **Start with a realistic goal.** Remember, 5 percent weight loss brings many health benefits. Lose that much weight and keep it off for at least six months before attempting to lose more.

2. **Be patient; aim to lose 1-2 pounds per week.** Know that initial weight loss will be greater than that, but be patient with modest

weight loss for the long haul. I remember Bert's goal was to lose two pounds weekly. Some weeks, he'd hit that goal; most weeks he didn't. To keep him from getting discouraged, I'd occasionally show him a graph of his weight-loss journey—over the course of time, his weight did steadily drop, and his health improved. (Note: Don't forget—1-2 pounds per week weight loss equals 52-104 pounds per year; a goal worth pursuing!)

3. **Find a food plan you like.** If you like your plan, whether it's low-fat or low-carbohydrate, you'll lose weight. Remember, you'll be eating like this for the rest of your life, with some modifications, to keep the weight off.

4. **Enlist support.** As I discussed in earlier chapters, you'll be much more successful in any behavior change with other people helping you along. Make sure family members know you're changing your eating habits and why, or join a weight-loss group in person or online. And *encourage compliments* from your supporters for positive behavior changes ("Great job exercising every day!"), *not reminders.*

5. **Monitor your eating habits**. Have a goal of getting an honest look at how much you're consuming. It helps to record food intake with an online program like MyFitnessPal. Whether you record online or with paper and pen, write down everything you eat—the amount, time, and calories. And look at why you're eating: Are you hungry or eating because you're sad, depressed, or celebrating? If you're bored, look for other ways to fill your time. If depression drives you to the fridge, try taking a walk instead.

6. **A deficit of 500 calories per day leads to weight loss of one pound per week.** This statement is true for most people

(1 lb. = 3,500 calories). The easiest way to do this is to combine cutting back on food intake with increasing exercise. For example: *Thirty minutes of most cardio burns 150 calories*. So you're looking to *cut back food intake by 350 calories per day* to reach your 500-calorie goal.

Here are some easy ways to start making that happen:

a. Cut back portion sizes. Use measuring cups and a food scale for a couple of weeks to get a true feel for the amount of food you're eating.

    •   Dropping from a 6-oz piece of meat to a 3-oz serving (recommended) saves over 200 calories.

    •   Replace regular dinner plates with salad plates or ones with a ten-inch or less diameter so you don't feel "cheated" with smaller portions.

b. Cut back on fats: One tablespoon of butter, margarine, mayonnaise, or most salad dressings equals 100 calories.

c. Cut back on high-calorie drinks.

    •   Most 16-ounce coffee drinks have 250+ calories

    •   A 20-ounce soda has 250 calories

    •   A 12-ounce can of beer for most brands has about 150 calories

    •   5 ounces of wine has 125 calories

    •   20 ounces of water has zero calories! (More on drinking water in Chapter 14.)

7. **Concentrate on foods that are low in calories but fill you up (low-caloric density).**

- Visually divide your plate into quarters: one quarter will be lean protein, one quarter whole grains, one half vegetables and fruit.

- Swap out desserts for tasty, in-season fruit.

8. **Eat enough protein.** Eating protein is especially important as you age.

   - Protein will help fight age-related muscle loss (sarcopenia) with its drop in metabolism.

   - Eat 10-20 grams of protein at breakfast to help stay fuller longer and fight off food cravings at night.

9. **Include meals plus snacks.** Eating small snacks with lean protein and complex carbohydrates can help preempt uncontrolled eating. The idea is to eat before you feel "starving" so you don't overeat at meals. Examples of such snacks are a whole-grain tortilla quesadilla (made with one tortilla), string cheese and a serving of whole-grain crackers, or peanut butter and one slice of whole-grain toast.

   - Make sure the snacks aren't *extra* calories; that is, eat small meals *and* small snacks.

10. **Exercise.**

    - Include strength training to help build and maintain lean muscle, which will support calorie burning by keeping your metabolic rate from tanking.

    - Include cardio to burn calories. (Remember, most thirty-minute bouts of cardio burn about 150 calories and provide many health benefits.)

    - If you can include an intense workout of either form, you'll continue burning calories for minutes to hours after you finish exercising because of EPOC (excess post-exercise oxygen consumption).

- Remember *not* to depend on exercise for weight loss; its better use is to help maintain pounds lost in the long run.

- Try using text messages to remind you to exercise (http://ohdontforget.com/).

11. **Boost your willpower.**[15]

- Repackage bulk food such as chips or crackers into smaller single serving bags.

- Reduce the size of dinner plates and glasses.

- Cover tempting foods in tinfoil.

- Make healthy food convenient and easily accessible.

Here are some additional success strategies from the thousands of weight-loss achievers/maintainers in the National Weight Control Registry: engaging in high levels of physical activity (approximately one hour per day); eating a low-calorie, low-fat diet; eating breakfast regularly; self-monitoring weight; and maintaining a consistent eating pattern across weekdays and weekends.

For aid in starting your own weight-loss program, check with your physician or health insurance program, or take cues from the DASH or Mediterranean diets.

EXERCISE

Select three of the above strategies that you feel you'll be successful at. Write a date when you will start them.

_____

_____

_____

SUMMARY

Losing extra pounds and keeping them off is critical for maintaining optimal health as we age. Of course, it's not an easy process; in fact, it's one that takes a lifetime commitment. But it can be achieved.

Remember to start with a small goal, 5 percent loss of your initial weight. And be honest with yourself—most people underestimate their food intake and overestimate their exercise minutes. Take stock of where you are right now, and choose a few small steps to get started. (Use SMART goals as we discussed in Chapter 3.)

Perhaps you can take another idea from the Blue Zones to help keep calories down: In Okinawa, residents practice "hara hachi bu," the 80 percent rule. This Confusian mantra is said before meals to remind people to stop eating when their stomachs are 80 percent full. It's a great way to stop mindless eating and keep calories down.

Be patient with yourself and know that any weight loss is healthful. And if you're currently at a healthy weight, do all you can to keep it that way. A study published in 2016[16] looked at 14,000 US individuals aged 50-89 over a fourteen-year period, focusing on three positive health behaviors, specifically:

- not obese (BMI less than 30)
- non-smokers (had smoked less than 100 cigarettes during their life)

- moderate alcohol drinkers (for men, less than fourteen drinks per week; for women, less than seven per week)

Compared to the general population, people with these three health behaviors lived 3-5 years longer, without disability (defined as no limitations in activities such as walking, dressing, bathing, getting out of bed, or eating). Not only was their longevity increased, but the added years were healthy ones.

So be mindful of your eating habits, keep moving, and celebrate weight-loss victories (with non-food rewards, of course!).

CHAPTER 14

GETTING CHUMMY WITH YOUR WATER BOTTLE

"I believe that water is the only drink for a wise man."

— Henry David Thoreau

In the previous chapters, I've focused a lot on food and mentioned water only briefly. However, water is an essential nutrient (you can't live without it), and our body's supply has to be replenished often. Assuming you have access to a clean source of water, the only question remaining is: How much is needed? The answer can be surprisingly complex.

So water deserves its own chapter. Let's plunge in!

SHE'S IN THE HOSPITAL FOR DEHYDRATION

The first time I heard this statement regarding my mother, I thought, "How can this be? She has access to water and other fluids, and she hasn't been feeling sick all that long." Luckily, the

ER personnel caught the problem right away, so she was hooked up to an IV by the time we got to the hospital.

Dehydration happens often, and it's become a familiar story with many older adults I know: a senior doesn't feel well and stops eating and drinking as much as usual. She becomes fatigued and confused. If nobody's paying attention, or if she lives alone, the lack of water can quickly become a life-threatening event.

We forget that water is a vital nutrient; life is simply not possible without it. Our bodies are about 50-70 percent water, and because we can't readily store or conserve it, we can only live on average three to five days without it.

Adequate water intake is important to help maintain normal body temperature, carry nutrients and oxygen to cells, and get rid of wastes—vital functions for living. In addition, water protects sensitive tissues, aids in digestion and absorption of food, and provides a moist environment for ear, nose, and throat tissues.

We lose water daily through breathing, perspiring, and urinating (a small amount is also lost with bowel movements). If we don't replace it, dehydration can set in, leading to urinary and kidney problems, seizures, and even death from low blood volume, which compromises the heart and other body systems.

Problems from dehydration start in the early stages of water deprivation—only a 1 percent decrease in body weight due to fluid loss (for example, if you weigh 150 pounds, your weight has dropped to 148.5 pounds.). At this point, most people start to experience thirst and begin losing the ability to regulate body temperature with exercise. Vague discomfort and loss of appetite start at a 2 percent loss. A 6 percent loss leads to a headache and stumbling. And a 10 percent loss (your weight is now 135 pounds) is life-threatening.[1]

Babies, older adults, and some people who are ill are most sensitive to dehydration. Many factors can cause dehydration: a lack of adequate water intake, extreme diarrhea and vomiting, excessive sweating and fever. For seniors, a decreased ability to conserve water and a reduction in thirst sensitivity intensify the problem. Chronic illnesses and medications also affect thirst. Lack of mobility can cause seniors to limit water intake.

And many health professionals believe thirst is *not* a good indication of hydration in elderly adults. In fact, "Because of their low water reserves, it may be prudent for the elderly to learn to drink regularly when not thirsty...."[2]

HOW MUCH IS ENOUGH?

Contrary to what you may believe, no official recommendation exists for *plain* water requirements. The most commonly repeated advice we all hear is, "Drink eight 8-oz glasses of water per day." As much as I have researched, there just is no hard science to support this statement. But it's become the mantra because it's easy to remember, and for most people, it fills the bill (more on that below).

Recommendations do exist for *total water* intake—that is, from *all beverages and foods*.

The National Academies of Sciences, Engineering, and Medicine recommend:[3]

- For women—approximately 2.7 liters (91 ounces) of *total* water each day

- For men—approximately 3.7 liters (125 ounces daily) of *total* water

- About 80 percent of total water intake comes from drinking water and other beverages (including tea, coffee, juices, sodas, and drinking water)

• The other 20 percent comes from food (think: watermelon, soup, spinach, etc.)

To put this in perspective, *if 80 percent of your fluid intake is from what you drink, that translates to the following amounts before any other factors are taken into account:*

• *72 ounces (9 cups) for women*

• *100 ounces (12.5 cups) for men*

(Another recommendation I've seen is based on how much you weigh: Drink at least a half-ounce of water per pound of body weight per day. For example, if you weigh 150 pounds, that would be 75 ounces or just over 9 cups.)

And like all wellness recommendations, check with your doctor to find out whether you have any special circumstances that influence your water requirements. But this at least gives us a number to aim for.

Note: These recommendations are for healthy people who are adequately hydrated. Young children, pregnant and lactating women, the elderly, and people with certain illnesses may have increased fluid requirements. In addition, exercise, weather, and elevation influence water requirements.

(As a side bar, when I was working as a school foodservice director, we were beginning to understand the importance proper hydration plays in helping youngsters be successful in academics. After all, the brain is about 75 percent water. Many teachers encouraged their students to keep water bottles with them, and schools were ensuring the availability of adequate, safe drinking water by upgrading water fountains and providing water-filling stations. On the other side of the age spectrum, every senior living facility I've visited has a constant supply of fresh, cool water available in large attractive containers for both residents and visitors.)

An unofficial recommendation I often pass on to people to monitor their hydration is the color of urine: If it's dark, you may be headed toward problems; if it's the color of lemonade (pale yellow), you're on track. However, many factors impact the color of urine (darker or discolored), including medical problems/illnesses, medications, and certain foods. But, in general, a light yellow is probably a good sign.

BUT LET'S JUST MAKE IT WATER, OKAY?

Here's why I recommend counting *only plain water*—maybe with sliced fruit or vegetables for added flavor—toward your water needs: I had a client last year who was overweight, inactive, and had type 2 diabetes. His drink of choice was Diet Coke. In fact, he'd drive to the local convenience store most mornings to bring home the largest container of soda he could buy. He'd refrigerate it and drink it all day long.

The reason this gentleman felt justified drinking so much diet soda was because his doctor told him it counted as part of his total water intake for the day. I doubted the veracity of this statement until I did more research on the subject. Turns out, as I stated earlier, *all* fluids do count.

But folks, let's get serious:

- Soda is full of sugar (16 tsp. per 20 oz.; that's 1/3 cup!), it's devoid of nutrients, and in my opinion, it's the poster child for unhealthy foods.

- Fruit juices, while containing vitamins and possibly added calcium, are equally as high in sugar, though the sugar is naturally occurring. Even pediatricians now recommend mothers do not give their babies and toddlers fruit juice. So dump juices and get the fiber, nutrients, and full feeling from whole fruits.

- Diet sodas have their own problems, being linked to weight gain and various health issues.

- Tea and coffee are great if they're "black," but how many of us doctor up our hot drinks with sugar and cream?

- Alcoholic drinks contain water, but their consumption inhibits a hormone that helps us conserve fluids when we start registering a shortage of available water. (In addition, somebody once told me: "Beer is for fans; water is for athletes!")

- And because so many Boomers and some seniors in this country are watching their weight and have access to potable water, H_2O is simply the overall best choice.

Adding weight to my opinion, a Beverage Guidance System was published a few years ago in the *American Journal of Clinical Nutrition*.[4] Its guidelines recommend drinking water as the preferred beverage to fulfill water needs, with the calories from all beverages being less than 10 percent of total calories for a 2,200 calories diet. That means less than 220 calories per day from non-water drinks, which is easily met by a soda, sports drink, coffee drink, or alcoholic beverage.

HOW TO GET ENOUGH

Many of my clients have difficulty drinking sufficient amounts of water. Here are ways to help you consume enough:

1. Buy a water bottle to easily track your intake. Most are 20-plus ounces, so aim for 3-4 full containers per day.

2. If you take medications, drink an 8-oz glass of water with each dose.

3. Because thirst is sometimes "felt" as hunger, drink water before eating.

4. Try different temperatures. Some people love icy cold water; I can down more at room temperature.

5. When you go to a restaurant, make water your go-to drink; add lime or lemon wedges.

6. Add sliced fruit or vegetables to flavor water without adding sugar or calories, and keep it refrigerated. Berries, citrus, and cucumbers make tasty additions.

7. Drink a glass before each meal. Bonus: This practice may help you eat less at mealtimes.

8. Set a timer to remind you to drink throughout the day.

Many older adults complain about getting up at night to urinate. If this is a problem, stop drinking water just after dinnertime; skew your intake heavily to the earlier part of the day.

EXERCISE

Come up with five specific ways you can up your water intake, working toward 9 (for women) or 12.5 (for men) cups per day.

1. _____

2. _____

3. _____

4. _____

5. _____

AND WHAT ABOUT WATER TOXICITY?

A few years ago, I remember hearing about a radio station that sponsored a water drinking contest to win a Nintendo Wii video game system. A woman who participated complained of a headache when she completed the contest, and she later died from water toxicity (drinking too much water). Although it seems implausible, this situation really does happen.

If we drink more water than our kidneys can get rid of, the level of some electrolytes in the bloodstream, especially sodium, can get too low. This imbalance leads to blurred vision and eventually death. But it's generally recognized that the intake of water would have to be excessive—*many* quarts per day (eight 8-ounce glasses = 2 quarts). Health professionals are mainly seeing water intoxication in athletes competing in events in which they overcompensate with water; that is, they drink more water than they perspire out.

Bottom line: While it's possible to drink too much water, it's not likely for most non-athletes.

(Note: Some people *must* limit their fluids. For example, people with kidney problems have to cut way back on water from all sources. Check with your doctor about recommended water intake.)

AND FILTERED WATER?

Most of us depend on tap water to fulfill our fluid requirements. But there have been concerns from time to time about possible contaminants in local water supplies. If you're worried about the safety of your water, you can request a copy of your water utility's annual water quality report. The Environmental Protection Agency does set regulatory limits for the acceptable amounts of certain contaminants in water.

Note: Do not depend on bottled water for water purity. The results of a four-year investigation published a few years ago concluded that up to 25 percent of bottled water is just plain tap water[5].

If you decide to purchase a water-filtering system, do your research. You don't need to spend thousands. Just find a product that will filter out contaminants, improve the flavor, be easy to install, and have a good warranty and customer service. And make sure it's certified by the NSF (National Sanitation Foundation).

SUMMARY

Water is vital for our survival. In fact, we can only live a few days without it. Water is a key transportation system in our bodies, responsible for delivering nutrients and oxygen, disposing of wastes, enabling important chemical reactions, protecting sensitive tissues, cushioning and lubricating joints, and aiding in the digestion and absorption of food.

Our bodies are 50-70 percent water. We lose water daily through breathing, sweating, and perspiration. A loss of water leads to dehydration, a potentially life-threatening condition, especially for babies, older adults, and people with illnesses. We eventually register "thirst" when we don't drink enough water. However, many experts believe we need to preempt the sensation of thirst and the resulting mild dehydration by drinking water throughout the day.

No known or defined requirement for water exists since it depends on several conditions, including illness, medications, exercise intensity, and elevation. Total water intake includes water from all fluids and foods, but *daily water needs are estimated at 9 cups/day for women and 12.5 cups for men.*

To reach these totals, we have to be creative and cognizant of our water intake. Using a twenty-plus-ounce water bottle and refilling it to monitor intake, plus varying flavors and water temperature are a few strategies to help meet your water needs.

It is possible, but not likely, to consume too much water.

And finally, if you don't want to drink a lot because you're concerned about getting up at night to urinate, concentrate on consuming the majority of your water by dinnertime.

CHAPTER 15

OPTIMIZING PROTEIN INTAKE

"Life goes faster on protein."

— Martin H. Fischer

In previous chapters, I've talked extensively about the importance of a plant-based diet. While eating less meat supports your wellness, I want to make sure one key nutrient isn't overlooked, and that's protein. It's misunderstood and often misused by people, but essential for health. And consuming enough at the right time of day will help you stay strong and independent as the years go by.

By helping build muscles or lean body mass (LBM), protein helps us stave off sarcopenia, the loss of muscle that starts after age thirty and results in a 3-5 percent decrease in LBM per decade. This loss is a serious problem for Baby Boomers and seniors, leading to falls and a loss of mobility, functional abilities, and independence.

The best way to fight sarcopenia is with strength training, supported by a proper diet. In particular, protein intake is key for maintaining and building muscle. In this chapter, I'll share what you need to know.

WHY DO I HAVE TO WORRY ABOUT PROTEIN AT MY AGE?

As I've mentioned before, I always analyze my clients' dietary intake. Over and over again, I've been surprised by their lack of protein intake. This was especially evident with Betty. A typical breakfast for her was cold cereal and some kind of sweet roll with coffee. She just wasn't very hungry in the morning, and with her limited mobility, she ate what was tasty and easy to grab. Lunch was soup or a salad. Like most Americans, she ate the majority of her protein at dinner.

After I explained to her the importance of protein throughout the day, we sat down and penciled out some acceptable meals and snacks for her.

Betty has typical eating habits for a person her age. While younger Americans tend to eat more protein than they need, older people often have the opposite problem, consuming less protein.

Protein is one of three macronutrients required in our diet (carbohydrates and fats are the other two)—it's needed in large amounts (grams versus milligrams or micrograms like vitamins and minerals) and it provides calories. It's been called the building block of life—every cell in our body contains protein. We need sufficient amounts to make enzymes, hormones, and other critical substances. Protein is present in muscles, bones, cartilage, skin, blood, hormones, and enzymes. It helps support wound healing and bolsters the immune system.

Our digestive system constantly breaks down protein from our diet into its amino acids components. These are then reassembled into the protein our bodies need for muscle-building, muscle repair, and the maintenance of key bodily functions.

WHAT AN ADEQUATE PROTEIN DIET LOOKS LIKE

Rick and Eva represent two ends of the protein-intake scale. Rick, a typical guy, loved to eat large servings of meat at dinner, while Eva's intake was small throughout the day. After Rick stopped rolling his eyes at me when I described the serving size of protein recommended for his dinner, and Eva understood the need to eat adequate amounts of protein all day long, we had some work to do to find eating patterns that worked for each of them.

Here are some official recommendations for protein intake:

- The Institute of Medicine of the National Academies develops the DRI (Dietary Reference Intake), which recommends 0.8 grams of protein per kilogram body weight.[1]
- The same agency recommends that 10-35 percent of calories should come from protein.[2]
- The USDA MyPlate recommends occupying only one-quarter of your meal plate with protein[3].

Bear with me for some numbers here:

Translating that first recommendation for you, let's say you weigh 150 pounds. The DRI is then about 54 grams of protein per day.

For ease of comparison, an eight-ounce glass of milk has 8 grams of protein, an ounce of meat has 7, and a serving of whole-grain bread has 3. So you can meet this requirement with two glasses of milk, 2 ounces of meat/protein at lunch, 3 ounces at dinner, and one whole-grain food.

A plate (read: "meal") with 3 ounces of protein, one whole-grain, two servings of non-starchy vegetables, one fruit, and one glass of low-fat milk is about 27 percent protein, well within the parameters set above for both the percentage of protein and the MyPlate recommendation.

However, two important points need to be made here:

• First, some research indicates that we actually need more protein as we age.[4] Older adults progressively lose muscle and are no longer very efficient at building it, so more good-quality protein, along with strength training, is critical. Some studies suggest that most people over sixty-five need 1.0-1.2 g. protein per kilogram body weight. This changes the above amount from 54 grams to 68-82 grams per day.

• Second, our bodies have a limited capacity to store protein for later use (whereas we are efficient at storing carbs and fats); we generally use protein as we eat it. If amino acids are not utilized soon after consumption to build protein, they can be transformed into carbohydrate (glucose).

So physiologically, if you eat large amounts of protein at night, and then sit down to watch TV, you don't need to build/replace/repair muscle. The protein is used elsewhere. And then, if you get up the next morning and exercise after a breakfast of cereal and fruit, the protein is gone from your overnight fast, so you might not have enough from your morning meal to fill your muscles' rebuilding needs for activity.

Therefore, *protein is best utilized if spread out evenly throughout the day.*

Spreading out our daily protein is especially critical as we age.[5] A new study looked at how protein is divided throughout the day to discover whether eating protein at all three meals would be beneficial. Researchers in Canada studied 1,700 healthy men and women, aged 67-84, for three years. The results: Those who consumed protein evenly at all three meals retained greater strength than those who ate most of their protein at dinner.

While this result is an observation of an association only, not a direct cause and effect, it does support other investigators who recommend an equal distribution of protein intake for older adults.

Do you consume adequate amounts of protein?

EXERCISE

Protein is found in soy products, dried peas and beans, nuts and nut butters, vegetables and whole grain products, and, of course, eggs, lean meat, fish, poultry, and dairy (including milk, cheese, cottage cheese, and yogurt). A variety of sources throughout the day will provide adequate protein. What foods do you eat that contain protein?

_____

_____

_____

_____

_____

ALSO HELPFUL FOR WEIGHT LOSS

Have you ever eaten a bowl of cereal for breakfast, only to feel hungry an hour or two later? This is a relatively common occurrence—a meal like cereal, lower in protein (and fat), is not very satisfying.

Protein provides satiety (a feeling of fullness) and is digested more slowly than carbohydrates, helping control hunger between meals. And if you eat healthy carbs (fruit, vegetables, or whole-grain products) with protein, the slower digestion can even out blood sugar and insulin levels.

Plus, as I've mentioned before, adequate protein, especially in folks over fifty, helps maintain lean body mass (LBM; read: muscle). If LBM goes down while you're dieting, there's a relative increase in the percentage of body fat. This changing dynamic is a death knell for weight loss because LBM burns more calories at rest than body fat does.

Dr. Freedhoff, in his book *The Diet Fix*, is adamant about including protein in all meals and snacks to maintain feeling full and stabilizing blood sugar and insulin levels. He recommends at least 20 grams of protein per meal and 10 grams per snack.[6]

So if you're one of the millions of adults trying to lose weight, an adequate amount of protein is critical, especially in the morning.

A DAY'S WORTH OF PROTEIN

When I work with clients, we strive to find 20 grams of protein for breakfast since the "sweet spot" for this nutrient seems to be *20-30 grams per meal*. Then we work on other meals. To most people, these are just numbers, so we are very specific in the foods that will work.

It's important to understand that our bodies require twenty amino acids (AA), building blocks of protein. We can make eleven of them from other dietary sources; nine are considered essential.

Foods that contain all nine are deemed complete proteins. Most foods in a vegan diet (i.e., no meat, dairy, or eggs), lack one or more essential AA, so it's important to eat a variety of these throughout the day.

For those folks eating a plant-based diet, high-quality non-meat proteins include soy/tofu, soy yogurt, lentils, pinto beans, quinoa, nuts, and seeds. Other sources include meat, dairy, and eggs.

So here's a primer on protein foods and amounts/sizes to meet your needs:

Meals

- I mentioned above that 1 ounce of a protein food contains about 7 grams of protein. So if you're depending on a purchased product for any meal or snack, simply check the Nutrition Facts label: 1) Look for the serving size. 2) Glance down toward the bottom of the label for the number of grams of protein per serving. This will tell you how much of the product to consume.

- A 3-ounce serving of most meats (21 grams of protein) is the size of your palm or a deck of cards.

- Foods you can use at breakfast for protein include eggs, cheese, cottage cheese, yogurt (dairy or soy), pinto beans, or even the entrée from last night's dinner.

Here's a sample menu with 20-30 grams of protein/meal

Traditional
Breakfast:
2 eggs scrambled with cheese (1/4 cup)
1 slice whole wheat toast
1 cup lowfat milk

Lunch:
Tuna salad (2 oz. tuna) on a bed of greens
1 serving whole-grain crackers
Greek yogurt, ½ cup
1 apple

Dinner:
Chicken, baked, 2-3 oz.
Quinoa, ½ cup
Zucchini or broccoli, steamed, ½ cup

Plant-based
Breakfast:
1 whole-grain English muffin, toasted
Peanut butter, natural, 2 Tb.
Yogurt, soy, 5-6 oz.
Sliced apple

Lunch:
Loaded baked potato (bake the night before and warm in microwave; add ½ cup garbanzo or black beans, 3 oz. plain soy yogurt,
chives, 1-2 Tb., soy-based "bacon bits")
1 serving whole-grain crackers
1 peach

Dinner:
Homemade burrito with 2/3 cup pinto beans and 1 oz. soy cheese
on whole-wheat tortilla
Brown rice, ½ cup
Green salad

Snacks
If you're dieting, strive to consume about 10 grams of protein at

mid-morning and mid-afternoon to help control your appetite. The following foods provide 7-10 grams of protein per serving, with 250 calories or less:

1. Hard-cooked eggs, 2 large eggs

2. Almonds, 1½ oz.

3. Protein powder (vegetarian is available), 1 scoop (Mix with lots of ice and your favorite fruit, fresh or frozen, or leafy greens.)

4. String cheese, 1 piece/28 grams

5. Peanut butter, natural, 2 Tb. Due to the high calorie content, be sure to measure out the two tablespoons of peanut butter at least once so you don't overindulge!

6. Yogurt, soy, 1 cup, or Greek, ½ cup, with fruit

PROTEIN BARS

Also known as meal replacement or snack bars, protein bars make an excellent, convenient between-meals food. Some of these products have up to 20-plus grams of protein per bar; others are closer to 10 grams. The former have more calories and are meant to replace meals. But the latter are easy to grab and store for quick snacks.

A plethora of protein bars are on the market. When searching for one to use as a snack, here are some guidelines to keep in mind:

• Look for ingredients containing "real" foods such as nuts and dried fruits

• 150-200 calories per serving

• 6-10 grams of protein

- 3-5 grams of dietary fiber
- Less than 3 grams of saturated fat
- Less than 10 grams of sugar (and watch for sugar alcohols such as maltitol, xylitol, or sorbitol, which can lead to bloating and diarrhea)

SUMMARY

Although most Americans get plenty of (or even too much) protein, consumption does tend to go down as we get older. This phenomenon may occur because of difficulty in chewing or cutting protein foods, or because of changes in taste due to medications. Unfortunately, the need for protein does not decrease. In fact, some experts believe our protein requirements are higher after age sixty-five.

A safe recommendation is 0.8 grams protein per kilogram of body weight per day for adults. For seniors, increase that to 1.0-1.2 grams per kilogram of body weight. No known benefit exists for consuming more than 2 grams of protein/kg body weight. (To calculate your weight in kilograms, take the number of pounds divided by 2.2.) In addition, excessive protein may cause nausea, weakness, diarrhea, and kidney problems. Check with your doctor to see whether you have any special needs regarding protein intake.

Because we don't store protein well, it's best spread out throughout the day. For most of us, that means eating a lot more for breakfast and a lot less at dinner.

With a little planning, it's easy to get 20-30 grams of protein per meal, even when eating a plant-based diet. And if you're trying to lose weight, adequate protein helps promote satiety and guard against insulin swings and food cravings later in the day. A 10-gram protein snack is also valuable for folks who are trying to control hunger throughout the day.

CHAPTER 16

KEEPING FALLS AT BAY

"Did you just fall down?"
"No, I attacked the floor!"

— Anonymous

A critical reason to eat adequate protein and engage in strength training is to take back your health and live an independent life as long as possible. That means staying safe and healthy into your seventies, eighties, and nineties. Along with managing chronic diseases, of key importance is minimizing falls, a major concern for older adults. Just the fear of falling causes many seniors to avoid being active altogether, further aggravating the possibility of growing weak and ill.

It's understandable that falling is a huge worry—an older adult is treated in the emergency room for a fall every eleven seconds, and one dies from a fall every nineteen seconds. And falls are a leading cause of injuries and death for folks aged sixty-five and older.[1] Broken bones (especially hips) lead to immobility and re-location to a nursing home—a one-way trip for many.

In this chapter, we'll look at the many situations that lead to falls, and what you can do to protect yourself or a loved one from this often fatal problem.

STOP WITH THE EXCUSES!

As I've said before, my mother was one of the main reasons I started my business. Her experiences were in many ways typical for older adults. For example, she fell more than once, both at her independent-care and assisted-care facilities. Although she had been given an alarm device to call for help, she didn't always wear it while in her apartment because she felt she only needed it when she left the facility.

Not true! In fact, this is a common misperception. Falls can happen anywhere. So right off the bat, let's look at five common myths about falls, debunked by the National Council on Aging:[2]

1. **Myth: I can avoid falls if I stay at home and limit activity.**

    Reality: More than half of all falls take place at home. My clients and my mother have all fallen more at home than in other locations. And by now, you know the importance of activity!

2. **Myth: Falling is a normal part of aging.**

    Reality: Falling is not a normal part of aging. We can all take steps to decrease the risk of falls with strength and balance exercises, taking care with medications, having our vision checked, and making our homes safe (details below).

3. **Myth: Falling happens to other people, not me.**

    Reality: Falls can happen to anyone; one in three older adults fall every year in the United States.

4. **Myth: Muscle strength and balance can't be regained.**

   Reality: While we do lose muscle strength as we age, it's never too late to start an exercise program—especially strength (resistance) training to begin restoring strength and flexibility to protect against falls.

5. **Myth: Using a cane or walker will make me more dependent.**

   Reality: When used properly, walking aids can help seniors maintain or improve mobility.

EXERCISE

What are your beliefs about falling? Do they just happen to "older people"? What can you begin doing today to reduce your risk of falling?

_____

_____

_____

_____

_____

IT'S BALANCE AND MUCH MORE

One day last winter, I went to work with Betty. I hadn't seen her for a couple of weeks because she'd been away visiting one of her daughters. When she opened the door, I was shocked to see fresh bruises on her face. I asked what happened, knowing what the answer would be. "I fell!" she said. She had been going downstairs and took a misstep while making a turn; down she went.

This is just one reason I've heard that causes my clients to fall. Others include tripping over cats, little dogs, or small children, getting up at night and falling over furniture, leaning on an unstable chair while putting on shoes, getting dizzy, reaching for a walker and missing it—the list goes on and on.

The point is: Many falls are preventable. They're not necessarily caused by "getting older" and "losing balance." With a little planning and diligence, hazards can be eliminated or minimized.

First, it's important to acknowledge that most older adults want to live on their own if they can. Many don't like to admit they have problems, so they don't ask for help. If you have a parent, grandparent, or older friend who lives alone, find a way to start a conversation with him or her about fall prevention. Maybe this person has fallen recently, or someone you both know has. Perhaps you could take advantage of changes in the person's medicine to discuss how it can cause dizziness. Or a segue into the discussion could be shopping with the loved one for new furniture or throw rugs. Take the opportunity to engage your senior to start looking for ways to stay on his or her feet.

Here are key areas to tackle when it comes to preventing falls:[3]

1. **Medications:** Find out whether any of the medicines you or a loved one are taking can cause dizziness, dehydration, or loss of balance. If this is the case, can they be replaced with other more benign drugs? What time of day is it best taken so as not to increase the risk of falling?

2. **Vision and hearing:** Many age-related eye problems de-

velop painlessly without symptoms. As a result, older adults have more difficulty seeing contrasting edges and tripping hazards. Chronic diseases such as diabetes and high blood pressure can lead to vision problems. The American Optometric Association recommends yearly eye exams once people reach age sixty.[4] Furthermore, studies show a correlation between hearing loss and balance problems with aging.[5] Hearing should be checked by an audiologist if there seems to be an issue in this area.

3. **Get enough sleep.**

4. **Limit alcohol:** Alcohol can affect balance.

5. **Environment:** Walk through your home or the home of an older loved one and look for these hazards:

   Floors: Get rid of throw rugs or purchase ones with non-slip backing; be sure the flooring is even with no holes or lifted areas; make sure you have a clear path through a room (move furniture if necessary); pick up all clutter and tape or move loose wires.

   Stairs: Be sure handrails are sturdy and available on both sides; clear clutter from area; make sure stairs are well-lit; repair broken steps.

   Bathrooms: Install hand-rails in shower/tub and next to toilet if needed; install non-slip rubber matting/strips in shower/tub; clear clutter off floor; get rid of throw rugs or purchase ones with non-slip backing; install night lights.

   Kitchen: To avoid over-reaching, place commonly used items in easy-to-reach areas. Avoid using step stools since they can be unsteady.

Bedrooms: Make sure a lamp is easily reached from bed; get out of bed slowly to avoid falling; if you use a walker, be sure it's placed safely near the bed and used properly.

A few additional safety tips:[6]

- Wear rubber-soled, low-heeled shoes that fully support your feet inside and outside; avoid going barefoot and wearing slippers.
- Keep emergency numbers in large print near each phone, especially near your bed.
- Put a phone near the floor in case you fall and can't get up.
- Think about wearing an alarm device to call for help if you fall.
- Install brighter light bulbs; florescent bulbs are bright and cost less to use.

In addition to managing your environment, engage in strength training, making sure your lower body and core stay as strong as possible.

It's worth repeating that when you exercise, evaluate your workout area for falls. Don't sabotage your safety and success. If exercising outside, find an area where the pavement is level and free of cracks. Be aware of curbs, holes in lawns, and the location of driveways; make sure you can cross the street before the light changes. If you plan to exercise indoors, find a room big enough for activity, and remove small carpets and electrical cords from the area. Exercises that help improve balance include yoga and Tai Chi.

EXERCISE

Is your home safe from falling?

Walk through your home with a list of areas: *floors, stairs, bathrooms, kitchen, bedroom, lighting, phones.* In which areas do unsafe conditions exist? Be sure to make changes as soon as possible to minimize your risk of falls.

_____

_____

_____

_____

_____

_____

_____

_____

_____

GETTING OFF THE FLOOR

More than once, a client has reported (with glee) that he or she has fallen, but was able to stand up easily without assistance! This is so important for anybody who lives alone. Sometimes, falls just happen, no matter how much planning there is, so it's critical to be strong enough to get off the floor as soon as possible. Like the commercials we see on TV, many older adults really do fall and then can't get up.

Keeping your legs and hips strong will help you stay up and get up. Exercises that help here are squats and lunges, or just getting out of a chair without using your hands to push off. Work with a physical therapist or personal trainer for exercises tailored to your needs.

If you do fall, try to use a sturdy coffee table or the edge of a sofa to help push yourself up. Or roll or crawl over to something you can hold for support to lift yourself. If no furniture is close by, try this method from the Geri-Fit program:[7]

- Get on all fours.
- Go backwards slowly and begin to straighten out the legs.
- Walk the hands backwards to the toes as the heels begin to touch the floor.
- Stand up slowly and carefully.

EXERCISE

1. Walk around your home and look for sturdy furniture, stairs, or other structures that can help you push yourself off the floor. List the sturdy objects that will aid you.

_____

_____

_____

_____

_____

_____

_____

_____

2. Next, practice getting up, both with this assistance and with-out. Become proficient at getting up without using a fixed object—this ability could save your life!

A FINAL NOTE ABOUT HIP FRACTURES

Finally, a major concern with falls is breaking a hip. For many older adults, a broken hip is literally the beginning of a down-ward spiraling cycle. So here's some information about hips and bones. Take a look at these sobering statistics from the CDC:[8]

- Each year over 300,000 older people—those sixty-five and older—are hospitalized for hip fractures.

- More than 95 percent of hip fractures are caused by falling, usually by falling sideways.

- Women experience three-quarters of all hip fractures.
    - o   Women fall more often than men.
    - o   Women more often have osteoporosis, a disease that weakens bones and makes them more likely to break.

- The chances of breaking your hip go up as you get older.

To decrease your risk of life-threatening hip fractures and to help keep bones strong, go back to Chapter 12 and reread the infor-mation about osteoporosis. Consume adequate amounts of cal-cium and vitamin D and engage in weight-bearing exercises such as climbing stairs, dancing, or jogging/fast walking. And keep your muscles strong by lifting weights.

SUMMARY

The fear of falling is huge among older adults. This fear often keeps people sedentary, further increasing their chances of developing chronic diseases and frailty. If you've fallen in the past, are concerned about falling, or have loved ones about whom you're worried, talk first to your or their healthcare provider. A geriatrician can help determine the cause or risk of falling, and refer you to helpful resources.

Engage other family members, friends, or neighbors who may live close by. They want to help seniors stay safe and independent. So enlist their support to help monitor the environment—both inside the house and outside—to make sure all safety concerns are addressed.

Look inside refrigerators and cupboards and take an honest assessment of foods available. Are you or your loved one consuming adequate healthy foods? If not, you may want to seek assistance from county agencies. In my home county of Riverside, California, we can dial 211 to receive information about a plethora of community services available.

Look for exercise programs to build balance, strength, and flexibility. Contact your local Area Agency on Aging or senior center for referrals. Find a program you like and take a friend.

And if you do go down, don't break your fall with your arms (this could lead to an upper body fracture). Instead, roll and try to land on your well-padded bum.

The bottom line regarding falls is that it is possible to reduce the risk of falling. Many resources are out there ready to help—you just have to reach out. Once you fall-proof your life, eat as well as you can and keep moving…safely!

CHAPTER 17

EATING AWAY FROM HOME—YOUR WAY!

"Shared dining fortifies us."

— Deng Ming-Dao

Now you're definitely ready to start on your wellness journey! You know your true "why," you've set up a support system, and you've figured out how to stay active and eat well. But life happens—you get tired, your friends invite you out for dinner, you go on vacation—and you start to get derailed.

In this chapter, we'll tackle the challenge of eating away from home, because you'll have to face this sooner or later, over and over again. And I'm well aware that food is much more than nutrition to most people. It's about great taste, celebrations, and sharing meals with loved ones.

So here are a few guidelines to protect your health while you go out and enjoy a great meal and social happening.

A NATIONAL PASTIME

I can still remember a married couple I met during one of my first jobs as a dietitian. He was a high school principal; she was a secretary. They attended an in-service about healthy eating for busy professionals. After the talk, the wife approached me with a huge challenge—they ate out almost every meal, most days of the week. They were both in their sixties and overweight. He had high blood pressure, she had type 2 diabetes.

I was shocked. With my knowledge of nutrition and lack of discretionary money at that early stage in my career, I couldn't fathom such an eating pattern. While this couple's dining out habits were extreme, it turns out they're similar to those of most Americans— we just don't love cooking at home any more. In fact, Americans buy a restaurant meal (lunch and dinner), snack, or drink about 4.5 times per week.[1]

And in 2015-2016, the average household spent nearly half of the money used for food on purchases away from home (43 percent). This number has been creeping up in recent years.[2]

AN EXERCISE IN EXCESS

When I go to a new restaurant, I always peruse the nutrition information looking for lower-calorie options. It's often difficult to find a regular meal that's under 500 calories. For this reason, some of my clients avoid dining out altogether.

But a recent article published in the *Journal of the Academy of Nutrition and Dietetics* found it's even worse than I thought. These researchers concluded that more than 90 percent of restaurants serve *entrées* that exceed the recommended calorie limit for a single meal. Meals, in general, average around 1,200 calories, with American, Italian, and Chinese food coming in at a whopping 1,495 calories.[3]

224

Considering the average woman eats about 2,000 calories per day, and men consume 2,500, you can see how quickly the pounds can start to add up!

In addition to calories, there are other health concerns when dining out—preparation style, freshness, type of added fat and salt, and huge portion sizes! In fact, portion sizes at restaurants and fast food establishments have doubled or tripled over the past twenty years[4]. For example:

- A typical bagel has grown from a 3-inch diameter to 6 inches.
- The average cheeseburger has gone up from 4.5 to 8 ounces.
- A medium bag of popcorn has exploded from 5 to 11 cups.
- A typical serving of soda has gone from 6.5 to 20 ounces.

These increases would add 1,595 calories to a daily energy intake or almost 600,000 calories (and dozens of pounds) a year!

A study published in the *International Journal of Obesity* looked at how those extra calories affect our health. Researchers found that people who eat six or more meals away from home per week had:[5]

- A higher body mass index (BMI)
- Lower levels of "good cholesterol" (HDL)
- Lower blood concentrations of certain nutrients

EXERCISE

Take a look at the past two weeks. How many of those fourteen days did you eat breakfast away from home? How many lunches and dinners did you consume at fast food establishments or restaurants? Now ask yourself why you ate that meal out—was it convenient, a time savings, a business meeting, or because of a lack of food at home? Be honest with yourself.

_____

_____

_____

_____

_____

WHAT'S A HUNGRY CONSUMER TO DO?

I would be remiss to avoid inserting here that one of the first things I advise my clients to do to improve wellness is to dine in as often as possible. It's cheaper and you can control the ingredients and healthfulness of the food. However, we enjoy eating meals away from home, and we will eat out often, so let's take a look at some best practices:

- Check the nutrition information on the menu. Restaurant chains with twenty or more locations are required to provide this. If you can find an item to eat as an entrée with 350-500 calories, go for it.

- Have a plan at mealtime and stick with it. If possible, look online for nutrition information and make a choice before you enter the restaurant. Then don't let other people's comments or choices influence your decision.

- Water is a great beverage of choice. You can ask for lemon or lime slices, go plain or sparkling, add ice or have no ice.

- Order off the kids' menu (easy at a fast-food restaurant but also possible at a sit-down chain—you can always ask). And take advantage of senior menus, which often have smaller portions.

- Split a meal two ways (or three).

- Instead of a main course, order an appetizer, soup, salad, or side dish; this is also a great option if you're going vegetarian.

- Ask to have your food customized: no sauces or added cheese, butter or sour cream; grilled protein foods instead of fried or breaded; find a substitute for fries or chips. In fact, a favorite breakfast order of mine reads as follows: omelet, no cheese; tomato slices instead of hash browns; fruit in place of bacon; whole-grain toast with butter on the side. It works!

- Skip dessert or ask for a clean spoon to share a bite of your dining partner's sweet indulgence.

- If all else fails, ask for a doggie bag to be brought to the table *with* your meal. Put half of your food in the container *before* you start to eat.

EXERCISE

Think of two favorite restaurants, one fast food and one sit-down. Now go back over the list above, or think of different strategies, and list at least five practices you will use to make meals healthier at each eating venue.

_____

_____

_____

_____

_____

_____

Some of my clients still work. They often skip breakfast altogether due to time constraints, or they just grab a coffee drink, breakfast bar, or bagel (these choices in general are high-sugar, low-protein, low-fiber; not the best choices for your health). If you work and eat meals and snacks at your workplace, the most important advice I can give you is to plan ahead. That's the only way you'll survive with a busy work schedule.

Having said that, here are ideas to help keep you fit for success:

1. Eat breakfast! This meal has its name for a reason: You've been fasting overnight, so it's time to put fuel into your body before you face the day, just as you would gas up your car.

2. Plan out your breakfast items the night before.

    • For example, if you're going to have oatmeal, mix together dry ingredients in a bowl and cover it with clear plastic. Leave the measuring cup close at hand, along with a spoon, so all you have to do in the morning is add water, cook, and enjoy.

    • If you're going to "pack" a breakfast—whether it's a hard-boiled egg, a protein bar (as a meal replacement, purchase one with 20 grams of protein), or peanut butter and a whole-grain English muffin—put everything together in one place where it's easy to grab before you leave for work.

3. Bring snacks. Include items that are both good sources of protein and dietary fiber to help keep you feeling energized longer.

    • Great ideas include: peanut butter and fruit, whole-grain crackers and peanut butter, Greek or vegan plain yogurt with fruit, a handful of nuts, and hummus and veggie sticks

4. Pack a lunch the evening before with last night's leftovers or a simple sandwich or salad with protein, fruit, and vegetables.

5. If you can't pack a lunch, follow the guidelines listed above for restaurant meals.

6. As I mentioned in previous chapters, get up and move every 30-60 minutes, and take advantage of breaks and lunch to engage in some sort of cardiovascular exercise.

EXERCISE

Think about a typical breakfast on a busy day. List 2-3 strategies you can use to enjoy a nourishing morning meal.

_____

_____

_____

WHAT ABOUT VACATIONS?

I worked with a couple last year who was planning a long vacation overseas. I had the opportunity to meet with them for several weeks before they left, hoping to help them get some good habits started. Before they left, I passed on these five strategies to enhance wellbeing while on vacation:

1. **Do some research:** Check for fitness opportunities your vacation locale might provide. Will you have access to a swimming pool or hotel gym? Can you take advantage of any stairways for climbing, or safe parking lots, community centers, parks, or indoor malls for leisurely walking?

    Make sure you have comfortable shoes and clothing. And plan accordingly for the weather—pack sunscreen, hats, sunglasses, insect repellant, and bottles for water.

And ask for a room with a small refrigerator.

2. **Pack your own "mini kitchen":** Nutritious food—don't leave home without it! If you'll be doing a lot of traveling, pack a small ice chest with fresh fruit and veggies, low-fat yogurt (don't forget plastic spoons), natural peanut butter, hummus, and bottles of water. Add whole-grain crackers or pretzels, unsalted or lightly salted nuts or even protein bars, and you should have plenty of sustenance to get from stop to stop.

3. **Think before you eat:** Bring snacks that can go into your hotel room refrigerator (low-fat or vegan yogurt and fruit) or do not require refrigeration (protein bars, nuts, peanut butter, and whole-grain crackers). Consume a protein source at each meal and at snacktime.

    Don't be hostage to breakfast buffets, fast food restaurants, and diners. It is possible to make healthy choices at these venues.

    *   *Breakfast*—Opt for fresh fruit, oatmeal, or whole-grain, low-sugar/high-fiber cold cereal, low-fat milk, yogurt, or eggs with whole-grain toast (light on the butter). Walk past the sweetened cereals, pastries, and breakfast meats.

    *   *Fast food restaurants*—Order a kid's meal, the smallest available burger, or a small "wrap." If you head for the salad bar, load up on the green leafies and other brightly-colored fruits and vegetables; limit starchy salads (pasta, potato); be sure to include some protein (hard-cooked eggs, kidney or pinto beans, or small amounts of grated cheese); and go light on salad dressings.

    *   *Family diners*—Enjoy a hearty meal, and follow the guidelines listed earlier in the chapter. In addition, watch the

free appetizers, limit added fats (butter, sour cream, salad dressing, gravy, sauces, and cream), and go sparsely on the salt (only after you've sampled the food).

4. **Make movement a priority:** Too much sitting time, while common with many vacations, wreaks havoc on your body—as I've said before. So when traveling, don't forget to engage your large leg muscles every hour or so. Stand when seat belts aren't required on the plane, and make frequent stops while driving.

   Once you reach your destination, find more ways to enjoy physical activity. Rent a bicycle or roller skates, or row a boat. Walk the downtown area to discover local food. Join nature treks whenever possible. And let the kid inside you run free! Soar on the swings, run through the sand, wiggle a hula hoop, or fly a kite.

5. **Bring your own exercise equipment:** Lightweight gear such as jump ropes and exercise tubing or bands are easy to pack and they provide great workouts. You can also find fitness apps like the 7 Minute Workout (https://7minuteworkout.jnj.com), which you can do in your room with no special equipment.

   So get packing, keep moving, and eat sensibly—bring home memories, not extra pounds!

EXERCISE

Do you have a vacation planned in the next few months? Take some time to contact the hotel or resort (online or by phone) to find out what sort of fitness amenities it provides. If none, is there a park, community center, or gym close by? What kinds of meals or foods does it offer? Are fresh fruit and water available 24/7? Specifically what types of foods are available at its breakfast buffet? If there's no restaurant or free breakfast, what types of foods does it sell? Can you get a room with a refrigerator, a microwave? Is there a healthful eating establishment close by?

Brainstorm the answers to these questions and more (go back to the guidelines above), and plan your next vacation with fitness and health in mind.

_____

_____

_____

_____

_____

_____

_____

_____

_____

_____

_____

SUMMARY

We Americans love to eat away from home. Whether it's break-fast with the family on the weekend, lunch at the ball park, or daily meals while on vacation, eating out is just part of our lives.

But, unfortunately, without judicious choices and planning, dining out is fraught with wellness land mines. These meals typically have excessive amounts of calories, sugar, fat, and sodium (salt). They can be low in dietary fiber and healthful phytochemicals from fruits, vegetables, and whole grains.

If you're trying to change your eating habits, don't deprive yourself while others are having a great meal. Instead, learn to make modifications. Employ any combination of the suggestions I've listed in this chapter, or any others that work for you. And remember, if there are no better options, enjoy a favorite food. Just remember these two caveats: Eat small amounts and splurge only occasionally.

CHAPTER 18

GIVING YOURSELF PERMISSION TO BE IMPERFECT

"Successful design is not the achievement of perfection but the minimization and accommodation of imperfection."

— Henry Petroski

As I mentioned in the previous chapter, dining away from home has become a regular part of our lives. The trick is to plan ahead, learn to make healthy modifications to your meal order, and enjoy food with family and friends. It's just as important to remember the key isn't to be perfect all the time, but to eat in a way that supports your wellness *most of the time*. If you "fall off the wagon" once in a while, don't dwell on it. Just get back on track as soon as you can.

And that brings me to the theme of this last chapter. Now that you have the components to build your enduring fitness, it's time to put all the information and effort into perspective. After all, Rome wasn't built in a day!

EXERCISE

Before we go further, remember back in Chapter 1 that I had you compile a list of diseases that run in your family. I asked you to put a checkmark next to conditions you believed you would inherit and could "do nothing about." Let's do that exercise again now and see whether after you've made your list, you've changed your mind about any of them.

_____

_____

_____

_____

_____

_____

IT'S A PROCESS, NOT A RACE

I ran into Jack at the gym a few weeks ago. I hadn't seen him for a year or so, and the first thing I noticed was that he looked thinner—much thinner. When I went up to congratulate him on his good work, he proceeded to complain about the slow rate of weight loss. In fact, he'd gone on a long bike ride the weekend before and hadn't lost any weight!

I often hear this sentiment from my clients. Unfortunately, we seek quick results when it comes to our health. I simply smiled at Jack and reminded him that he didn't get where he was overnight. I recommended he plot out his weight loss on a graph. Watching the line representing "pounds" drop down over time is always a powerful reminder of the positive changes you are making.

More importantly, it's a way to see that changes occur *over time*. Developing new habits is not easy, but it is possible. It's about creating a mindset to support a *lifestyle change*, not trying to lose weight before you jump on a cruise ship or run off to your forty-year reunion. Don't think in terms of a finish line. Ask anybody who has lost a significant amount of weight and kept it off, or who has turned around prediabetes, and that person will tell you it's something he or she works on all the time.

I also like to remind people that time goes on regardless of the choices you make. Summer will come after spring; you'll be a year older when the calendar dictates. So you might as well do something positive for yourself during that time. Do you want to gain weight again next holiday season, get another lecture from your doctor about your blood chemistry at a follow-up appointment, or notice more weakness in your legs when you go on vacation in a few months? Or do you want to have started lifestyle changes to take back your health? It's your choice; you're at the helm.

EXERCISE

Where do you want to see your health a year from now? Do you want to be off some of your medications, have the energy to play with your grandchildren again, and be able to get up from the floor if you fall? List at least three goals.

1. _____

2. _____

3. _____

Now sit across from an empty chair and pretend your "successful self" from twelve months in the future is facing you. What lifestyle changes will he or she congratulate you upon accomplishing? What will your future self scold you on for having been too impatient about? Remember, he or she is in the future and knows what's happened this year as you've been accomplishing your goals.

(I realize this exercise may sound silly, but please bear with me—this can be a powerful exercise if done with an open mind.)

_____

_____

_____

_____

_____

_____

_____

_____

_____

THE 80/20 RULE

Nobody's perfect all the time. We're humans, not machines. Life happens, and the most we can do is to put our best plans in place, anticipate the problems that will occur, and move forward.

Margaret is a perfect example of how this works. She is still very independent and lives with her husband, who is not quite as fit as she. Margaret does her own shopping and food preparation, especially important to support her vegetarian lifestyle. Her goal when she met me was to lose a little weight and become more active, getting back into an exercise "habit."

But she's also a social butterfly—she loves enjoying food with friends and family. Every week, I'd ask Margaret what plans she had for the weekend, and we'd talk about potential roadblocks to her fitness program. Then we'd review what happened the following Monday.

In general, she was successful in dropping a little weight over time. And she reestablished a walking and gym program. But there were weeks when we'd laugh about the foods she couldn't resist (she had a real weakness for sweets)—especially when somebody dropped off goodies at the agency where she volunteered her time. Margaret was able to keep her long-term goal in mind and didn't beat herself up over her occasional transgressions.

She followed the 80/20 rule—staying the path most of the time, and getting back on her plan the next day.

EXERCISE

With your goals in mind, think about what's coming up in the next twenty-four hours. Don't think long-term; just concentrate on the decisions you'll need to make *immediately*. What problems are likely to block your forward movement? Are there ways you can mitigate the damage—eat dinner before visiting friends one evening, not walk past the cookie plate every time you get up to answer the phone, make sure you get your walking and strength training in, even if you did eat that dessert?

List one issue you'll face today that might send your fitness plans into a tailspin, and make some decisions that embrace the 80/20 rule.

_____

_____

_____

_____

_____

_____

_____

_____

_____

GIVE YOURSELF A BREAK

We are all our own worst enemies! And I include myself in that statement. We constantly beat ourselves up for not being perfect. While we'd be the first to tell another person to "chill out" with the self-criticism, we can rarely turn that mirror around and take our own advice. In fact, I've heard that 60-80 percent of the 50,000-70,000 thoughts we have each day are negative.

But it's time to admit that perfect isn't real. At many of the business meetings I attend, I hear the following phrase, "Completion, not perfection." Truly take this to heart—just work toward your goals and don't stumble over your imperfections. Remember, your body responds to the long-term habits and lifestyle changes you're making, not the occasional hiccup.

So be kind to yourself. Give yourself permission to fail once in a while. Missteps are just normal human behavior. Don't get upset, and don't throw weeks of work out the door because you feel bad about one slip-up. Life is complicated and uncertain; just make the best of it and keep your chin up (as I used to tell my kids).

Have that yummy ice cream cone when the urge hits; savor every mouthful, and then *just move on*. (This is an example of mindful eating—paying close attention to the moment and accepting your feelings, not trying to change them.)

AND FINALLY, CELEBRATE!

When my clients do a good job reaching their goals, I urge them to celebrate. Of course, I don't mean with a piece of cheesecake or a hot fudge sundae. I challenge them to come up with relevant rewards.

When thinking about rewards, keep these guidelines in mind:

1. **Break goals into small steps.** Then reward yourself when you accomplish each of these steps. If your long-term goal is to drop twenty pounds, and your new weekly goal is to walk ten minutes twice a day, celebrate that small (but significant) accomplishment.

2. **Make rewards relevant.** I'd love to buy myself an arrangement of fresh flowers as a way to acknowledge an accomplishment, while my husband would rather spend an hour at the bookstore perusing the latest science fiction books. What makes you shine?

3. **Don't forget that a reward doesn't have to be something you spend money on.** It can just be appreciating how good you feel as a result of reaching your goal. Maybe you have more energy now, you can zip up your pants a little easier, or you can get out of a chair without relying on pushing yourself. Feel proud and victorious; pat yourself on the back.

4. **Concentrate on the positive and don't "punish" the imperfections.** Research shows rewarding good behavior is more effective than berating yourself for doing something wrong.

5. **Celebrate with significant people in your life.** We talked earlier about the importance of having a team to support your efforts. Allow these folks to share in your successes as you make positive gains.

EXERCISE

Take the time now—before you get busy changing your life—to list out rewards you will give yourself. You'll be celebrating small successes, so you'll need lots of ideas. Here are some thoughts: going to a movie; enjoying a manicure, pedicure, or massage; spending time at the bookstore or library; visiting your local museum; buying an updated piece of fitness equipment (maybe a fitness tracker?); or taking a stroll in nature.

Come up with ten relevant, motivating rewards.

_____

_____

_____

_____

_____

_____

_____

_____

_____

_____

SUMMARY

In this last chapter, I've given you permission to write yourself a hall pass once in a while. Making behavioral changes leading to a healthier life is not easy; that's why we are where we are in terms of our national and global wellbeing (or lack thereof). So be kind and forgive yourself as needed. The worst thing you can do is get upset because you overate or skipped exercising for the week and then just throw in the towel.

Remember that you are on a journey that will last forever, in terms of your life. So don't try to race to the finish line. Make a decision to start someplace, now! Tell loved ones what you're doing and ask for support. If needed, seek professional advice from your healthcare provider, a health coach, a registered dietitian, a physical therapist, or a certified personal trainer.

Don't strive for perfection; you'll just cause yourself aggravation. Instead, follow your plan 80 percent of the time, and when you blow it, just accept that life happens; get back with the program and move on. Stop being your own worst enemy and catch any negative, defeating self-talk that can lead you back to the sofa or dessert menu.

And, finally, celebrate successes, big and small. It's the best way to reinforce positive behavior changes you're making and keep yourself motivated for the long haul. Be sure rewards are relevant and immediate, and share triumphs with others who are important in your life.

This bears repeating: Take a good look at yourself and decide to take action. It's your health, your independence, and your life. Start with small goals, and start *today*. Best wishes for your success and wellness!

LIVING YOUR BEST LIFE NOW

That's it! I've given you the best lifestyle strategies to outsmart Mother Nature. Now that you've finished my book, what actions are you going to take? What goals are you going to set? Which health professionals or important people in your life are you going to reach out to for help in your journey? What books are you going to read, and which seminars are you going to attend? What changes in your life are you going to make?

Before you add this book to the "I've finished these" row on your bookshelf, I challenge you to take action! Now it's your turn to take the lead in achieving the healthy, independent life you desire and deserve. Think of it this way—knowledge is not power until it's applied. You can read all the best-selling health and fitness books in the world (and there are a lot of them), but if you don't make it personal, if you don't start applying the information to make critical lifestyle changes, you will not live out your years with the quality life you're looking forward to.

So here we go. Please use this book as it is intended—as your wellness resource. Take all the information in it that's relevant to your life; now, grab a pen or pencil and list on the lines below the ten actions you commit to taking within the next ninety days.

_____

_____

_____

_____

_____

_____

_____

_____

_____

_____

In this book, you learned to become the leader in your own health journey. You've put in place a support system and grasped the importance of moving every day, concentrating on a plant-based diet, adding both strength training and cardio to your exercise program, and attacking chronic diseases. I've given you tips to age with strength and independence, to drop a few pounds and keep them off, to avoid falls, to be successful eating outside the home, and much more.

The good news is that if you follow the strategies and wisdom offered in this book, you will achieve your self-leadership roadmap to optimum health and build your own enduring fitness.

Now that you've read my book, I encourage you to contact me. Please tell me what you liked, or disliked, about it. Because the fields of both fitness and nutrition are so dynamic, I will be sure to write further editions of this book, and your comments will help me make improvements. But more importantly—so I can help you—please share a bit about yourself, your challenges, and your obstacles. To better assist you, I would like to offer you a complimentary, no-obligation 30-60-minute consultation via phone, Skype, or FaceTime, or even in person (if geography allows).

My email address is lisa@enduringfitness4u.com and my cell phone is (951) 533-2612. Please email or text me with your name and your time zone so we can schedule your complimentary consultation and I can see how I can help.

And finally, I want to leave you with an uplifting message—words of wisdom I found on Facebook from a ninety-year old:

- Life isn't fair, but it's still good.
- When in doubt, just take the next small step.
- Life is too short not to enjoy it.
- Save the things that matter.
- Make peace with your past so it won't screw up your present.
- It's okay to let your children see you cry.
- Don't compare your life to others'. You have no idea what their journey is all about.
- Take a deep breath; it calms the mind.
- Get rid of anything that isn't useful. Clutter weighs you down in many ways.
- It's never too late to be happy. But it's all up to you and no one else!

I wish you much success on your wellness journey. May you live your life with the quality and self-sufficiency you seek, and may you attain your enduring fitness.

Lisa Harris

SPECIAL REPORTS

HEALTHY FOODS

As you now know, our bodies change in a number of ways as a result of aging. Perhaps the most noticeable is a decline in caloric need as activity levels and metabolism shift downward, along with muscle mass.

So while we need the same amount of nutrients (more in some cases), we need to get them with less calories—foods that deliver the biggest bang for our buck. Unfortunately, our parents often purchase items that are easy to prepare, chew, and swallow, and that provide comfort (think: desserts). Often little attention is paid to nutrition.

Here are steps you can take to help improve the nutritional quality of your parents' diets:

1. **Snoop.** When visiting mom or dad, see what foods are in the cupboard and refrigerator. Do you see any whole-grain pasta, brown rice, whole-grain/lower-sugar cereals? Are there any dairy products in the refrigerator; how about fresh fruits and vegetables? Are any products out of date?

2. **Encourage water intake**. Have mom or dad purchase a 20-ounce water bottle to track the amount consumed.

3. **Go shopping with them.** Check out the deli section of your local grocery store; many have prepared salads and entrées (watch sodium); split a rotisserie chicken, which can be cut into portions and frozen for future meals.

4. **Pack snack-sized foods.** Make sure your parents have healthy

snacks readily available such as whole-grain crackers, fresh fruits, baby carrots, nut or protein bars (keep the sugar as low as possible, with high dietary fiber), plain Greek or soy yogurt (add own fruit), string cheese, and cottage cheese.

5. **Encourage lower-cost, high-quality protein sources.** Sources can include eggs, cottage cheese, canned tuna, and dried or canned beans.

6. **Economize by encouraging them to buy frozen fruits and vegetables.** Frozen produce is often a better choice than fresh because it's packed at peak season, it's lower in cost, and leads to less waste.

7. **Become a stellar health advocate.** Ask doctors to check for nutritional-related deficiencies including B vitamins (especially B12 and folate), vitamin D, and iron; a bone density scan (DEXA) will help diagnose osteoporosis/osteopenia, which may affect nutritional needs.

8. **Encourage a 2-3 oz serving of protein at each meal, especially breakfast.**

9. **Invite Mom/Dad over for meals.**

PHYSICAL ACTIVITY

In my business, I've learned folks in their eighties definitely have mitigating circumstances that limit their mobility (diabetes, nerve damage, arthritis, heart disease). But the unfortunate truth is that often older folks spend time sitting because they spend time sitting. That is, they're not immobile because they're growing older, but they're growing older because they're immobile.

And when movement grinds to a halt, so does quality of life. Seniors begin to experience falls, dependency on others for day-to-day tasks, and depression—which often leads to even less activity.

If you're the primary caregiver for your parents, here are three tips you can use to help them remain independent for as long as possible. (Note: Check with your parents' primary healthcare provider to make sure there are no health problems requiring special attention.)

1. **Watch for signs of increasingly sedentary behavior**. Is your mom or dad sitting in a favorite recliner every time you visit? Is the TV always on? Is the extent of their activity using their thumbs on the remote control? Do you seldom see them walking from room to room or even standing tall? Are they starting to need help with stairs, getting in/out of chairs or cars, or carrying groceries?

2. **Help find local activities.** Help your parent/s locate an exercise program. While there are fitness opportunities online or on DVDs, encourage your loved ones to get out and mingle with others. Check the local senior center (senior centers often offer

fitness classes for free or reduced costs), the YMCA, your local parks and recreation, city-run classes, or a local junior college. Programs must include strength training, not just movement. Pushing/lifting body weight, light dumbbells, and resistance tubing are absolutely vital to stop the decline in muscle tissue and strength. You may hear a lot of excuses, so research transportation and try to find your mom or dad a buddy.

3. **Be a loving child, not an enabling one.** When it comes to encouraging movement, be insistent. Seniors hate being treated like children by their own children. I know—because they tell me! So don't do everything for them. Set high expectations. Ask Mom and Dad to come up with a reasonable, measurable goal they can work on each week, and check back with them consistently. For example, attending a strength-training class twice a week, buying a pedometer and increasing steps by 100 weekly, or decreasing television viewing thirty minutes. If all else fails, take your parents to visit a local assisted-care community (say you're just checking out facilities and costs). Maybe after seeing all the people using walkers, electric scooters, and wheelchairs, they'll be more motivated to take control of their own wellbeing!

A RECIPE FOR HEALTHY GRANDCHILDREN

Many of us are taking care of Mom or Dad, and helping our children by babysitting grandkids on a regular basis. Although it may be tempting to plop little ones down with a bag of chips in front of a TV, cell phone, or computer tablet so you can have time to yourself, don't do it!

Grandparents can play a key role in helping little ones develop healthy habits. Here are a few guidelines to keep in mind the next time you babysit:

GET THEM AWAY FROM THEIR SCREENS

The American Academy of Pediatrics (AAP) came out with recommendations for media use in 2016.[1] According to AAP, the average child today spends seven hours per day in these sedentary behaviors, which can lead to attention problems, school difficulties, eating and sleeping disorders, and obesity. Here's a summary of their recommendations:

- For children younger than eighteen months, avoid use of screen media other than video-chatting. Parents of children 18-24 months who want to introduce digital media should choose high-quality programming, and watch it with their children to help them understand what they're seeing.

- For children ages 2-5, limit screen use to one hour per day of high-quality programs. Parents should co-view media with children to help them understand what they are seeing and apply it to the world around them.

- For children ages six and older, place consistent limits on the time spent using media, and the types of media, and make sure media does not replace adequate sleep, physical activity, and other behaviors essential to health.

- Designate media-free times together, such as dinner or driving, as well as media-free locations at home, such as bedrooms.

- Have ongoing communication about online citizenship and safety, including treating others with respect online and offline.

Here are some other ways you can help:

- It's important for children to spend time on outdoor activities, reading, hobbies, and using their imagination in free play. We did it when we were kids, so grab a Frisbee, a paintbrush, or sheet (to make an indoor tent, of course!) and play with them!

- Encourage your grandchildren to engage with you in daily chores. They can help sort or fold laundry, carry light bags of groceries or individual items into the house, or scoop out dry pet food for your furry companions.

- Be creative; show kids how to complete the task properly, and let them build self-confidence while promoting healthy habits.

AVOID FOOD FIGHTS!

When it comes to food, remember, you're the responsible adult! Kids may request food they see advertised on TV, but you're in control of two key parameters: *when* food is available, and *which* foods are available. Then kids control how much they eat.

Here are some guidelines from ChooseMyPlate.gov to help develop healthy eating patterns in kids:

- Focus on the meal and each other. Children mimic your be-haviors, so model good eating habits and a willingness to try new foods.

- Offer a variety of healthy foods. Do this often; then let the kids choose how much they eat.

- Be patient! Children are notoriously slow eaters. (I should know—I was a school foodservice director for almost twenty years!) Encourage them to finish eating during mealtime, and save leftovers for snacks (if appropriate). Don't expect little ones to accept new foods right away—offer frequently and give just a taste at first.

- Let children serve themselves. Teach them to take small amounts initially, with more coming as needed!

- Let kids help in meal planning, shopping, and preparation, as much as possible.

TEN FITNESS MISTAKES YOU *DON'T* WANT TO MAKE

When I start working with Baby Boomers or older adults, they're amazed by the information I provide! To me, as both a certified personal trainer and registered dietitian, it's important to give accurate and valuable advice. And whether it's correcting bad (and potentially unsafe) form when lifting weights or reshaping eating habits, I've seen a lot of fitness mistakes over the years.

I've put together a list of the ten most common errors I see; be careful not to make these!

1. **Thinking exercise alone will lead to significant weight loss.** Many people start working out at the gym expecting to lose weight. While physical activity does burn calories, the numbers are not significant for noticeable weight loss. Most experts agree that weight loss is actually 75-80 percent what goes into your mouth.

2. **Giving up on exercise when no weight loss occurs.** While exercise isn't the greatest help for weight loss (it is, however, a major key to weight maintenance), physical activity does reduce the risk of thirty-five harmful conditions and life-threatening diseases, including premature death. The bottom line: Don't stop moving! Your health and wellbeing are depending on you.

3. **Doing the same exercises all the time.** In order to build muscle size and strength, it's important both to change up your

routine and gradually increase the load. For example, do cardio before strength training once in a while, or vice versa. And most importantly, if you can easily perform twelve reps of one exercise, increase the weight by 10 percent.

4. **Exercising heavy every day.** It's critical to give your muscles forty-eight hours to recover before challenging them again. That means you can do upper body one day, lower the next, or both upper and lower every other day.

5. **Ignoring diet altogether.** In addition to promoting weight loss as mentioned above, eating the proper amount of protein (see #8 below), at the proper times, promotes muscle gain and maintenance for a stronger body—one able to function easily with all the activities of everyday life, including balance. Diet is also critical for blood sugar control, blood pressure, and a host of other health conditions.

6. **Not thinking about water.** Consuming enough water is important while exercising. Adequate fluid intake transports nutrients to cells and waste products away from them, and it keeps muscle cells working properly. Don't depend on your thirst—drink the number of ounces of water equal to half your weight, or enough to keep your urine the color of lemonade (light yellow).

7. **Avoiding carbohydrates.** Many people think they need to avoid carbohydrates to be fit. Not true. Muscles use stored carbohydrates (glycogen) for energy, which must be replaced after exercising. And the brain uses carbohydrates exclusively for energy. The key is to select the right carbs, not to avoid all of them!

8. **Eating too much protein at night.** While we can use them for

energy, protein calories are best used for muscle growth and repair, especially as we grow older. Unfortunately, our bodies have limited capacity to store excess dietary protein from a single meal. So if you consume a large steak for dinner and don't pick up your dumbbells until tomorrow, that protein isn't contributing to muscle growth. It's best to eat equal amounts of protein at breakfast, lunch, and dinner.

9. **Concentrating exclusively on cardio.** Cardio is great for your physical and mental health. But weight training is arguably more important. It helps build and maintain muscles to keep us from falling and losing our independence, contributes to an increase in the rate of calorie burning, and helps strengthen bones.

10. **Not asking for help.** Whether you're in a gym or the doctor's office, it's important to reach out to trained professionals. Your own healthcare professionals, registered dietitians, physical therapists, and personal trainers can help you get more fit, without injuring yourself, or wasting your time and money.

MORE HERBS, LESS SALT = FLAVOR + HEALTH!

I've picked up on a new trend lately—my husband and I were out to dinner recently when we noticed there were no salt and pepper shakers or packets anywhere to be seen! Of course, we didn't need them because the food was so fresh and flavorful, but this reinforced a healthful concept I teach in my fitness business—decreasing salt intake.

One way to reduce your salt is to replace salt with herbs. This food preparation method has become so popular there's even a National Day for it: August 29 is More Herbs, Less Salt Day. This recognition day encourages us to take a simple step to eat with wellness in mind, through the use of herbs in home-cooked dishes in place of salt.

THE GOOD...

Herbs are nature's medicine cabinet, in use since ancient times. More recent research has confirmed that herbs contain compounds called polyphenols—powerful antioxidant and anti-inflammatory agents. These tiny miracle workers may help protect against conditions such as cancer, diabetes, and heart and brain disease. Some herbs also contain vitamins A, C, and K, bestowing further health benefits.

While fresh herbs give foods a clean, springlike taste, they must be eaten within a few days of cutting. To enjoy herbs for a longer time, consider using the dried versions, which also spice up foods and add health benefits. The drying process actually concentrates the polyphenols and flavors, plus it makes them easy to store, and they will stay good for about a year.

THE BAD...

Most of us eat too much salt, and as a result, we consume too much sodium, the true culprit in this twin-component chemical structure (salt = sodium + chloride). In fact, Americans eat about 50 percent more than the recommended amount of sodium. Sodium is a required nutrient, needed to control blood pressure and blood volume, as well as nerve and muscle action. But too much sodium can lead to extra fluid in the body, high blood pressure, heart attack, and stroke.

Consuming homemade foods without added salt is a great start to a healthy eating pattern since approximately 75 percent of our sodium comes from processed foods and restaurant meals.

AND EASY WAYS TO GET RID OF THE UGLY!

Here are seven ways to reduce salt, and add more herbs to your diet:

1. Encourage people to taste food before they add salt.
2. Use a dash of seasoned salt (for example, Lawry's) in place of salt; it has one-third less sodium than salt. Or even better, use a non-salt product such as Mrs. Dash.
3. Don't put salt on the table unless requested.
4. Add cilantro and parsley to green salads.
5. Add dill, rosemary, or tarragon to entrées.
6. Add dried thyme to cooked vegetables.
7. Add fresh parsley or dill into boiled or mashed potatoes.

FOODS HIGH IN DIETARY FIBER

Use this chart to help reach the recommended daily amounts of fiber: men, 38 grams per day, women, 25 grams per day.

Fruits	Serving Size	Total fiber (grams)
Raspberries	1 cup	8.0
Pear, with skin	1 medium	5.5
Apple, with skin	1 medium	4.4
Banana	1 medium	3.1
Orange	1 medium	3.1
Strawberries (halves)	1 cup	3.0
Figs, dried	2 medium	1.6
Raisins	1 oz. (60 raisins)	1.0
Vegetables		
Artichoke, cooked	1 medium	10.3
Green peas, cooked	1 cup	8.8
Broccoli, boiled	1 cup	5.1
Turnip greens, boiled	1 cup	5.0
Brussel sprouts, cooked	1 cup	4.1
Sweet corn, cooked	1 cup	4.0
Sweet potato, baked or boiled	1 small	4.0
Potato, with skin, baked	1 small	3.0
Tomato paste	¼ cup	2.7

Carrot, raw	1 medium	1.7
Grains, cereal, and pasta		
Spaghetti, whole-wheat, cooked	1 cup	6.3
Barley, pearled, cooked	1 cup	6.0
Bran flakes	¾ cup	5.3
Oatmeal, instant, dry	½ cup	4.0
Popcorn, air-popped	3 cups	3.5
Rice, brown, cooked	1 cup	3.5
Bread, rye	1 slice	1.9
Bread, whole-wheat	1 slice	1.9
Legumes, nuts, and seeds		
Split peas, cooked	1 cup	16.3
Lentils, cooked	1 cup	15.6
Black beans, cooked	1 cup	15.0
Baked beans, vegetarian, canned, cooked	1 cup	10.4
Sunflower seed kernels	¼ cup	3.9
Almonds	1 oz. (23 nuts)	3.5
Pistachio nuts	1 oz. (49 nuts)	2.9
Pecans	1 oz. (19 halves)	2.7

SAMPLE MENU WITH >30 GRAMS OF DIETARY FIBER

(grams of fiber shown in parentheses)

Breakfast	Snack
Oatmeal, ½ cup cooked (4)	Apple, with skin, 1 (4.4)
Strawberries, fresh, ½ cup (1.5)	Crackers, whole grain, 1 svg
Milk, 1%, 1 cup	String cheese, 1 oz.
Greek yogurt, vanilla, nonfat, 5.2 oz	
Lunch	
	Snack
Bean burrito on whole-wheat burrito (4)	Orange, 1 (3.1)
Carrot, raw, med, 1 (1.7)	Almonds, 1 oz. (3.5)
Banana, 1 (3.1)	
Dinner	**Snack**
Chicken, bbq, 3 oz.	Popcorn, air-popped, 3 cups (3.5)
Broccoli, ½ cup cooked, (2.6)	
Sweet potato, small, 1 (4)	
Salad w/olive oil dressing	

ADDITIONAL RESOURCES

Academy of Nutrition and Dietetics (AND)
http://www.eatright.org

Alzheimer's Association
https://www.alz.org

American Bone Health
https://americanbonehealth.org

American Cancer Society
https://www.cancer.org

American College of Sports Medicine
http://www.acsm.org

American Council on Exercise (ACE)
https://www.acefitness.org

American Diabetes Association
http://www.diabetes.org

American Heart Association
http://www.heart.org/HEARTORG/

Arthritis Foundation
http://www.arthritis.org

Blue Zones
https://bluezones.com

Geri-Fit Strength Training for Older Adults
https://www.gerifit.com

International Osteoporosis Foundation
https://www.iofbonehealth.org

National Council on Aging
https://www.ncoa.org

National Institute on Aging
https://www.nia.nih.gov/health

National Osteoporosis Foundation
https://www.nof.org

OsteoStrong
http://osteostrong.me

Silver and Fit
https://www.silverandfit.com

SilverSneakers
https://www.silversneakers.com

WORKS CITED

Chapter 1

1   https://www.ncoa.org/news/resources-for-reporters/get-the-facts/healthy-aging-facts/

2   https://health.clevelandclinic.org/2017/06/how-americans-feel-about-living-to-be-100-infographic/

3   http://www.journalofaccountancy.com/news/2016/oct/americans-fear-running-out-of-retirement-money-201615242.html

4   Ratey, John J. Spark: *The Revolutionary New Science of Exercise and the Brain.* New York: Little, Brown and Company, 2008.

5   https://www.johnhancockinsurance.com/life/life-expectancy-tool.aspx

6   Wan, H. et al. *65+ in the United States: 2005 Current Population Reports.* Washington, DC: US Census Bureau, 2005. p. 23-209. http://www.census/gov/prod/2006pubs/p23-209.pdf

7   https://www.cdc.gov/aging/pdf/State-Aging-Health-in-America-2013.pdf

8   Hoffman, C., Rice, D., and Sung, H. Y. "Persons with chronic conditions: their prevalence and costs." *JAMA.* 276.18 (1996):1473-1479. https://jamanetwork.com/journals/jama/article-abstract/410506?redirect=true

9   https://journalistsresource.org/studies/government/healthcare/elderly-medical-spending-medicare

10 https://www.cdc.gov/aging/pdf/State-Aging-Health-in-America-2013.pdf

11 https://www.ncoa.org/news/resources-for-reporters/get-the-facts/healthy-aging-facts/

12 https://www.care.com/c/stories/10329/the-hiring-caregivers-guide-the-cost-of-caregivers/

13 http://www.aarp.org/ppi/info-2015/caregiving-in-the-united-states-2015.html

14 http://www.retirementthrudesign.com/resources/weekly-newsletter/114-what-baby-boomers-worry-about

15 https://www.acefitness.org/blog/6429/genetics-or-lifestyle-which-matters-more-for-men-s

16 Northrup, Christine. *Goddesses Never Age*. Carlsbad, CA: Hay House, 2015.

17 http://www.drnorthrup.com/goddesses-never-age-best-years-ahead/

18 http://www.who.int/chp/chronic_disease_report/part1/en/index11.html

Chapter 2

1 Bryant, Cedric X. and Daniel J. Green, eds. *ACE Personal Trainer Manual*. 4th ed. San Diego, CA: American Council on Exercise, 2010.

2 Ibid.

3 https://www.psychologytoday.com/blog/flourish/201210/happiness-is-risky-business

Chapter 3

1 Bryant, Cedric X. and Daniel J. Green, eds. ACE Personal Trainer Manual. 4th ed. San Diego, CA: American Council on Exercise, 2010.

2 http://jamesclear.com/habit-stacking

3 Price, Derrick. "Habit-Based Coaching: Finding the Right Cues to Reap Rewards." Fitness Journal. June 2017, p. 42-49.

4 https://www.acefitness.org/acefit/fitness-fact-article/3279/gathering-support-for-your-active/

5 https://www.supertracker.usda.gov

6 http://www.myfitnesspal.com

7   https://health.usnews.com/health-news/diet-fitness/fitness/slideshows/fitness-excuses?slide=2

Chapter 4

1   "McDonald's, Ubereats Will Take It To Go." *Press Enterprise.* Friday, May 19, 2017.

2   Levine, James A. *Get Up: Why Your Chair Is Killing You and What You Can Do About It.* New York, NY: St. Martin's Griffin, 2014.

3   Morris, J. N. et al. "Coronary heart disease and physical activity of work." Lancet. 262.6796 (1953): 1053-1057.

4   Biswas, Aviroop, et al. "Sedentary Time and Its Association With Risk for Disease Incidence, Mortality, and Hospitalization in Adults: A Systematic Review and Meta-analysis." http://annals.org/aim/article/2091327/sedentary-time-its-association-risk-disease-incidence-mortality-hospitalization-adults.

5   http://www.who.int/dietphysicalactivity/factsheet_inactivity/en/

6   Levine, James A. *Get Up: Why Your Chair Is Killing You and What You Can Do About It.* New York, NY: St. Martin's Griffin, 2014.

7   Levine, J. A. "Non-exercise activity thermogenesis (NEAT)." *Best Pract Res Clin Endocrinol Metab.* 16.4 (2002): 679-702.

8   http://care.diabetesjournals.org/content/diacare/suppl/2016/12/15/40.Supplement_1.DC1/DC_40_S1_final.pdf

9   Troiano, R. P. et al. "Physical activity in the United States measured by accelerometer." Med Sci Sports Exerc. 40 (2008): 181-8.

10 Kelly Bowden-Davies, M.Sc., Institute of Aging and Chronic Disease, University of Liverpool, U.K.; Minisha Sood, M.D., endocrinologist, Lenox Hill Hospital, New York City; May 17, 2017, presentation, European Congress on Obesity, Porto, Portugal.

Chapter 5

1   Buettner, Dan. *The Blue Zones: Lessons for Living Longer From the People Who've Lived the Longest.* Washington, DC: National Geographic Society, 2008.

2   Farmer, B. et al. "A vegetarian dietary pattern as a nutri-ent-dense approach to weight management: an analysis of the national health and nutrition examination survey 1999-2004." *J Am Diet Assoc.* 111.6 (2011): 819–27. DOI: http://dx.doi.org/10.1016/j.jada.2011.03.012.

3   Snowdon, D. A., Phillips, R. L. "Does a vegetarian diet reduce the occurrence of diabetes?" *Am J Public Health.* 75.5 (1985): 507–12. DOI: http://dx.doi.org/10.2105/AJPH.75.5.507.

4   de Lorgeril, M. et al. "Mediterranean diet, traditional risk factors, and the rate of cardiovascular complications after myocardial infarction: final report of the Lyon Diet Heart Study." Circulation. 99.6 (1999): 779–85. DOI: http://dx.doi.org/10.1161/01.CIR.99.6.779.

5   https://www.ncbi.nlm.nih.gov/pmc/articles/PMC5466938/

6   http://www.bmj.com/content/357/bmj.j2241

7   Estruch, Ramón et al. "Primary Prevention of Cardiovascu-lar Disease with a Mediterranean Diet." *N Engl J Med* 368 (2013): 1279-1290. DOI: 10.1056/NEJMoa1200303.

8   Luciano, Michelle, et al. "Mediterranean-type diet and brain structural change from 73 to 76 years in a Scottish cohort." *Neurology.* 88.4 (2017): 449-455.

9   Yang, Y. et al. "Association Between Dietary Fiber and Lower Risk of All-Cause Mortality: A Meta-Analysis of Cohort Stud-ies." *Am J Epidemiol.* 181.2 (2015): 83-91.05.

10 https://www.ncbi.nlm.nih.gov/pubmed/27252308

11 https://health.gov/dietaryguidelines/2015/resources   2015-2020_Dietary_Guidelines.pdf

Chapter 6

1 Webb, Densie. "Phytochemicals' Role in Good Health." Today's Dietitian.15.9 (2013): 70.

2 https://health.gov/dietaryguidelines/2015/resources/2015-2020_Dietary_Guidelines.pdf

3 http://www.aicr.org/assets/docs/pdf/brochures/eat-well-to-reduce-your-cancer-risk.pdf

4 Centers for Disease Control and Prevention. "Adults Meeting Fruit and Vegetable Recommendations—United States, 2013." Morbidity and Mortality Weekly Report. 64.26 (2015): 709-713.

5 Aune, Dagfinn et al. "Fruit and vegetable intake and the risk of cardiovascular disease, total cancer and all-cause mortality—a systematic review and dose-response meta-analysis of prospective studies." Int J Epidemiol. February 22, 2017. DOI: https://doi.org/10.1093/ije/dyw319.

Chapter 7

1 https://www.marketplace.org/2013/03/12/life/big-book/processed-foods-make-70-percent-us-diet

2 Barr, S. B. and J. C. Wright. "Postprandial energy expenditure in whole-food and processed-food meals: implications for daily energy expenditure." Food Nutr Res. 54 (Jul 2, 201054). doi: 10.3402/fnr.v54i0.5144.

3 https://www.cdc.gov/salt/pdfs/role_of_sodium.pdf

4 Wansink, B. "Change Their Choice! Changing Behavior Using the CAN Approach and Activism Research." Psychology & Marketing. 32 (2015): 486–500. doi:10.1002/mar.20794

5 Sotos-Prieto, Mercedes, et al. "Association of Changes in Diet Quality with Total and Cause-Specific Mortality." N Engl J Med. 377 (2017): 143-153. DOI: 10.1056/NEJMoa1613502

Chapter 8

1. https://www.acefitness.org/acefit/fitness-fact-article/3293/energize-your-life-with-strength/

2. Shiroma, Eric J. et al. "Strength Training and the Risk of Type 2 Diabetes and Cardiovascular Disease." Med Sci Sports Exerc 49.1 (2017): 40-46.

3. O'Connor, P. J., Herring, M. P., and Caravalho, A. "Mental health benefits of strength training in adults." *American Journal of Lifestyle Medicine.* 4.5 (2010): 377–96.

4. Bickel, C. S., Cross, J. M., and Bamman, M. M., "Exercise dosing to retain resistance training adaptations in young and older adults." *Med Sci Sports Exerc.* 43.7 (2011): 1177-87. doi: 10.1249/MSS.0b013e318207c15d.

5. https://www.cdc.gov/nchs/data/nhis/earlyrelease/earlyrelease201705.pdf

Chapter 9

1. https://www.cdc.gov/nchs/fastats/exercise.htm

2. https://health.gov/paguidelines/guidelines/summary.aspx

3. http://www.exerciseismedicine.org/assets/page_documents/eim-fact-sheet-2015.pdf

4. https://www.cdc.gov/physicalactivity/basics/pa-health/index.htm

5. http://www.exerciseismedicine.org/assets/page_documents/eim-fact-sheet-2015.pdf

6. Ratey, John J. Spark: The Revolutionary New Science of Exercise and the Brain. New York: Little, Brown and Company, 2008.

7. http://www.sciencedirect.com/science/article/pii/S0091743517301470

8. http://www.cell.com/cell-metabolism/fulltext/S1550-4131(17)30099-2

9. http://orthoinfo.aaos.org/topic.cfm?topic=a00418

10. https://www.acsm.org/docs/brochures/high-intensity-interval-training.pdf

Chapter 10

1. Hoffman, C., Rice, D., and Sung, H. Y. "Persons with chronic conditions: their prevalence and costs." JAMA. 276.18 (1996): 1473-1479.

2. King, Dana E. et al. "The Status of Baby Boomers' Health in the United States: The Healthiest Generation?" JAMA Internal Medicine. 173.5 (2013): 385-386.

3. https://www.heart.org/idc/groups/ahamah-public/@wcm/@sop/@smd/documents/downloadable/ucm_480086.pdf

4. http://www.heart.org/HEARTORG/HealthyLiving/Make-the-Effort-to-Prevent-Heart-Disease-with-Lifes-Simple-7_UCM_443750_Article.jsp#.WYtXwq3Myu6

5. https://www.cdc.gov/diabetes/pdfs/data/statistics/national-diabetes-statistics-report.pdf

6. http://www.who.int/mediacentre/factsheets/fs312/en/

7. http://www.hopkinsmedicine.org/news/media/releases/small_survey_most_primary_care_physicians_cant_identify_all_risk_factors_for_prediabetes

8. http://www.nejm.org/doi/full/10.1056/NEJMoa1504347#t=article

9. https://www.niddk.nih.gov/about-niddk/research-areas/diabetes/diabetes-prevention-program-dpp/Pages/default.aspx

10. http://care.diabetesjournals.org/content/diacare/suppl/2016/12/15/40.Supplement_1.DC1/DC_40_S1_final.pdf

Chapter 11

1 https://www.cancer.gov/about-cancer/understanding/statistics

2   https://www.cancer.gov/about-cancer/causes-prevention/ge-netics/genetic-testing-fact-sheet

3   https://seer.cancer.gov/archive/csr/1975_2009_pops09/re-sults_single/sect_01_table.11_2pgs.pdf

4   https://www.cancer.org/healthy/eat-healthy-get-active/acs-guidelines-nutrition-physical-activity-cancer-prevention/guidelines.html

5   http://www.who.int/features/qa/cancer-red-meat/en/

6   Lauby-Secretan, Béatrice et al. "Body Fatness and Cancer—Viewpoint of the IARC [International Agency for Research on Cancer] Working Group." *N Engl J Med.* 375 (2016): 794-798. DOI: 10.1056/NEJMsr1606602

7   http://www.alz.org/facts/

8   https://www.rush.edu/news/diet-may-help-prevent-alzheimers

9   Ratey, John T. *Spark: The Revolutionary New Science of Exercise and the Brain.* New York: Little, Brown and Company, 2008. p 10.

10 https://www.ncbi.nlm.nih.gov/pubmed/26819457

11 http://www.thelancet.com/journals/lancet/article/PIIS0140-6736(17)31363-6/abstract

12 https://www.cancer.gov/about-cancer/understanding/statis-tics and http://www.alz.org/facts/

13 https://www.alz.co.uk/research/statistics

Chapter 12

1   http://www.arthritis.org/about-arthritis/understanding-arthri-tis/arthritis-statistics-facts.php

2   https://www.iofbonehealth.org/facts-statistics

3   http://www.arthritis.org/about-arthritis/understanding-arthri-tis/arthritis-statistics-facts.php

4   https://www.cdc.gov/vitalsigns/arthritis/

5   http://www.arthritis.org/living-with-arthritis/arthritis-diet/anti-inflammatory/the-arthritis-diet.php

6   https://nccih.nih.gov/health/glucosaminechondroitin#hed2

7   https://www.nof.org/patients/what-is-osteoporosis/

8   Jaquish, J. "Multiple-of-bodyweight axial bone loading using novel exercise intervention with and without bisphosphonate use for osteogenic adaptation." *Osteoporosis International*. 24.4 (2013): 198.

Chapter 13

1   http://www.nytimes.com/2013/06/19/business/ama-recognizes-obesity-as-a-disease.html.

2   https://www.health.harvard.edu/staying-healthy/exercise-and-aging-can-you-walk-away-from-father-time

3   https://stateofobesity.org/healthcare-costs-obesity/ A review of obesity-related economic studies

4   https://www.world-heart-federation.org/resources/diet-overweight-obesity/

5   http://www.obesity.org/content/weight-diabetes

6   https://www.cancer.gov/about-cancer/causes-prevention/risk/obesity/obesity-fact-sheet

7   https://www.sciencedaily.com/releases/2008/05/080507105556.htm

8   Jiang, L. et al. "The relationship between body mass index and hip osteoarthritis: a systematic review and meta-analysis." *Joint Bone Spine*. 78 (2011): 150-5. [PubMed]

9   Jiang, L. et al. "Body mass index and susceptibility to knee osteoarthritis: a systematic review and meta-analysis." Joint Bone Spine. 79 (2012): 291-7. [PubMed]

10 Rena R. Wing, et al. "Benefits of modest weight loss in improving cardiovascular risk factors in overweight and obese individuals with type 2 diabetes." *Diabetes Care*. 34(7) (2011): 1481–1486.

11   Knowler, W. C. et al. "Reduction in the incidence of type 2 diabetes with lifestyle intervention or metformin." *N Engl J Med.* 346.6 (2002): 393-403.

12   www.nwcr.ws

13   Johnston, B. C. et al. "Comparison of weight loss among named diet programs in overweight and obese adults: a meta-analysis." *JAMA.* 312.9 (2014): 923-33. doi: 10.1001/jama.2014.10397.

14   Freedhoff, Yoni. *The Diet Fix: Why Diets Fail and How To Make Yours Work.* New York, NY: Harmony Books, 2014.

15   Kompf, Justin. "Self-Regulation Strategies for Barriers to Weight Loss." *ACSM Health & Fitness Journal.* 21. 6 (2017): 27-32.

16   Mehta, N. and Myrskylä, M. "The Population Health Benefits of a Healthy Lifestyle: Life Expectancy Increased and Onset of Disability Delayed." *Health Aff (Millwood).* (2017 Jul 19). pii: 10.1377/hlthaff.2016.1569. doi: 10.1377/hlthaff.2016.1569. [Epub ahead of print] https://www.ncbi.nlm.nih.gov/pubmed/28724530

Chapter 14

1   Wardlaw, Gordon M. and Smith, Anne M. *Contemporary Nutrition.* 9th ed. New York: McGraw-Hill, 2013. p. 354.

2   Popkin, Barry M., D'Anci, Kristen E., and Rosenberg, Irwin H. "Water, Hydration, and Health. Nutr Rev. 68.8 (2010): 439-458.

3   http://nationalacademies.org/hmd/~/media/Files/Activity%20Files/Nutrition/DRI-Tables/9_Electrolytes_Water%20Summary.pdf?la=en

4   Popkin, BM et al. "A new proposed guidance system for beverage consumption in the United States." *American Journal of Clinical Nutrition*, 83 (2006): 529.

5   https://www.nrdc.org/stories/truth-about-tap

Chapter 15

1   http://www.nationalacademies.org/hmd/~/media/Files/Activity%20Files/Nutrition/DRI-Tables/8_Macronutrient%20Summary.pdf?la=en)

2   http://www.nationalacademies.org/hmd/Reports/2002/Dietary-Reference-Intakes-for-Energy-Carbohydrate-Fiber-Fat-Fatty-Acids-Cholesterol-Protein-and-Amino-Acids.aspx

3   http://hnrca.tufts.edu/myplate/files/MPFOA2015.pdf

4   Bauer, J. et al. "Evidence-based recommendations for optimal dietary protein intake in older people: A position paper from the PROT-AGE Study Group." *J. Am. Med. Dir. Assoc.* 14 (2013): 542–559. doi: 10.1016/j.jamda.2013.05.021.

5   http://ajcn.nutrition.org/content/106/1/113.abstract?related-urls=yes&legid=ajcn;106/1/113

6   Freedhoff, Yoni. *The Diet Fix: Why Diets Fail and How To Make Yours Work.* New York, NY: Harmony Books, 2014.

Chapter 16

1   https://www.ncoa.org/news/resources-for-reporters/get-the-facts/falls-prevention-facts/

2   https://www.ncoa.org/healthy-aging/falls-prevention/preventing-falls-tips-for-older-adults-and-caregivers/debunking-the-myths-of-older-adult-falls/

3   https://www.ncoa.org/wp-content/uploads/cksafety.pdf

4   https://www.aoa.org/patients-and-public/good-vision-throughout-life/adult-vision-19-to-40-years-of-age/adult-vision-over-60-years-of-age

5   Koh, Da Hyun, Lee, Jong Dae, and Lee, Hee Joong. "Relationships among hearing loss, cognition and balance ability in community-dwelling older adults." J Phys Ther Sci. 27.5 (2015): 1539-1542. Published online 2015 May 26. doi: 10.1589/jpts.27.1539.

6   https://www.ncoa.org/wp-content/uploads/cksafety.pdf

7   Geri-Fit Strength Training for Older Adults. Instructor Training Manual. Geri-Fit Company: 2013.

8   https://www.cdc.gov/homeandrecreationalsafety/falls/adulthipfx.html

Chapter 17

1   https://www.zagat.com/b/the-state-of-american-dining-in-2016

2   https://www.bls.gov/news.release/cesan.nr0.htm

3   Urban, Lorien E. et al. "Energy Contents of Frequently Ordered Restaurant Meals and Comparison with Human Energy Requirements and US Department of Agriculture Database Information: A Multisite Randomized Study." *Journal of the Academy of Nutrition and Dietetics.* 116.4 (2016): 590–598.

4   https://www.nhlbi.nih.gov/health/educational/wecan/news-events/matte1.htm

5   http://www.nature.com/ijo/journal/v39/n5/full/ijo2014183a.html

Special Reports, A Recipe for Healthy Grandchildren

1   https://www.aap.org/en-us/about-the-aap/aap-press-room/pages/american-academy-of-pediatrics-announces-new-recommendations-for-childrens-media-use.aspx

ABOUT THE AUTHOR

LISA TERESI HARRIS is an author, professional keynote speaker, health and wellness coach, and an award-winning entrepreneur. A registered dietitian since 1978, she started her second career as a fitness professional at age fifty-nine. Currently, she's the owner of Enduring Fitness 4U, where she provides senior exercise classes and in-home fitness training and nutrition coaching, as well as virtual programs.

Lisa was inspired to start helping others realize their best lives after battling her own incurable autoimmune disease and then witnessing her mother's strength start to deteriorate in her eighties.

Lisa's goal—her undying "why"—is to empower folks to live out their lives with as much strength and independence as possible. Through her coaching and speaking, she's inspired hundreds of people to get stronger and live longer.

She lives with her husband, Terry, and their cat in Temecula, California, close to her two children and three grandchildren.

ABOUT ENDURING FITNESS 4U SERVICES

If you're a Baby Boomer trying to delay the effects of aging, or an older adult struggling to remain self-sufficient, you're not alone!

Lisa Teresi Harris is a fellow Boomer. She lives in the Temecula area of Southern California, and she knows that growing older is unavoidable. However, we now have a large body of evidence leading us to an encouraging conclusion: With active intervention, we can maintain our quality of life well into our later years.

But don't go it alone—there's just too much confusing information out there!

Lisa works closely with her clients to help them overcome the challenges. Together, they create an individualized program of personal training and nutrition guidance to support the lifestyle changes for *the client's* specific wellness needs!

To learn how Lisa can support your wellness needs, visit her website or text her with your name, time zone, and the best time to schedule a 30-60-minute, no-obligation consultation by phone, Skype, or FaceTime.

And grab her free e-book, *7 Top Fitness Myths Debunked*, at http://enduringfitness4u.com/7-fitness-myths/.

www.EnduringFitness4U.com
www.BuildingYourEnduringFitness.com
(951) 533-2612
lisa@EnduringFitness4U.com

BOOK LISA TERESI HARRIS TO SPEAK AT YOUR EVENT

As a registered dietitian and certified personal trainer, Lisa Teresi Harris is passionate and enthusiastic; she engages her audiences with inspiration, education, and practical tips. She provides tools attendees can use right away to enjoy greater health and well-being.

From eating strategies to hands-on strength-training exercises, Lisa empowers audiences to move toward living a healthier life.

A sought-after fitness professional, author, and speaker, Lisa firmly believes you have the power to add quality and longevity to your life, no matter the age, through physical activity and nutritious foods—and she can show audiences how! Lisa's talks are appropriate for all audiences—keynotes, breakout sessions, conferences, retreats, associations, and forums. Her content can be easily customized to your particular group or industry; just ask!

Contact Lisa by phone or email to schedule a complimentary pre-speech phone interview:

Lisa@EnduringFitness4U.com
(951) 533-2612